I dedicate this book to all victims and sufferers of MRSA.
Past. Present. Future.

Maggie Tisserand

Medical Disclaimer

This book is not intended as a substitute for professional help. If your symptoms persist, you should consult a medically qualified practitioner.

AROMATHERAPY VS MRSA

ANTIMICROBIAL ESSENTIAL OILS TO COMBAT THE SUPERBUG

MAGGIE TISSERAND

THECLARITYPRESS

Published by
THE CLARITY PRESS
11 High Street,
Upper Gravenhurst,
Bedfordshire, MK45 4HY, UK

First published by The Clarity Press September 2011
10 9 8 7 6 5 4 3 2 1

**British Library Cataloguing in Publication Data. A catalogue record for
this book is available from the British Library.**

ISBN 978-0-9568941-0-6

Book design: Mark McClung
Bembo NT 9 - 20 and Tahoma 9 - 20
Back Cover photograph copyright Luci Tisserand

Printed and bound in Great Britain by MPG Biddles Ltd. King's Lynn

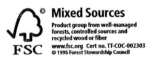

© **Mixed Sources**
Product group from well-managed
forests, controlled sources and
recycled wood or fiber
www.fsc.org Cert no. TF-COC-002303
© 1996 Forest Stewardship Council
FSC

THECLARITYPRESS
www.theclaritypress.co.uk

Contents

Acknowledgements   vii

Introduction   ix

Part One   **MRSA**

Chapter 1   MRSA – World View   3

Chapter 2   MRSA – Human Stories   13

Chapter 3   MRSA in Animals   21

Chapter 4   Evolution of MRSA   31

Chapter 5   Microbiology Explained   39

Part Two   **Antimicrobial essential oils**

Chapter 6   Tea tree   47

Chapter 7   Manuka   57

Chapter 8   Thyme   69

Chapter 9   Further Research with Essential Oils   79

Chapter 10   Other Ways to Combat MRSA   89

Part Three   **Appendices**

Appendix I   Facts & Figures   97

Appendix II   Reasons for Resistance   100

Appendix III   Risk Factors   102

Appendix IV   Before Going into Hospital   106

Appendix V   Essential Oils   114

Appendix VI   Wound Care   120

Appendix VII   Extra Reading   126

Appendix VIII   Organisations   128

Resources   Products   133

Resources   Services   138

Glossary   141

References   146

About the Author   159

Also by Maggie Tisserand

Aromatherapy for Women
Essential Oils for Lovers
The 14-Day Aromabeauty Plan
Stress: The Aromatic Solution
The Magic and Power of Lavender★
★*co-authored with Monika Junemann*

Acknowledgements

I owe a great deal to everyone involved with the creation of this book, which has been two and a half years in the making. The writing of the book came about as a direct consequence of the previous five years of microbiology research, and my grateful thanks go to the following:

John Smart, Professor of Pharmaceutical Sciences and Head of the School of Pharmacy and Biomolecular Sciences, and Geoffrey Hanlon, Professor of Pharmaceutical Microbiology, Pharmacy and Biomolecular Sciences, University of Brighton, for welcoming my project; Dr Jonathan Caplin, Department of Environment & Technology and Dr Iain Allan, Department of Pharmacy and Biomolecular Sciences, who, under the supervision of Professor Hanlon, conducted many months of microbiology trials; and lastly, to all of the Business Development Managers I have worked with over the years at the University of Brighton.

For the publication of this book, my deepest thanks go to Lizzie Pollock, a long term friend and supporter who set up The Clarity Press in order to bring this book to market. Thanks also to Lizzie for her editing skills and for working tirelessly with me over the past eighteen months. I thank Mark McClung for his creativity and expertise in book design, Harry McDowell for proof reading, Lucy and Jonathan Rouse for their input with some of the appendices.

Many people have been instrumental in the bringing together of this book, and my thanks go to: Tony Field, founder of the MRSA Support Group for his consistent championing of my research; Derek Butler of MRSA Action for taking my phone calls; to Emma, Bill, Dave, Tom, Julie and Hazel from the MRSA Support Group, who in 2004, responded to my call for volunteers; to Sylla Hanger-Shepherd from Tampa, Florida, for her support at the early stage of book writing and for introducing me to MRSA sufferers in North America; and to all the survivors of MRSA who have spoken to me at length about their encounter with a very frightening disease.

Contributions to the book have been generously given and I give special thanks to Valerie Edwards-Jones, Professor of Medical Microbiology, Manchester Metropolitan University for contributing Microbiology Explained. Special thanks also go to Dr Jonathan Caplin for contributing The Evolution of MRSA. I also would like to thank Jill Moss of the Bella Moss Foundation for providing additional information on zoonotic disease for chapter five.

For helping me understand the complexities of colonisation I thank Sylvie Hampton, Tissue Viability Consultant at the Wound Healing Centre, Eastbourne; and Andrew Kingsley, Clinical Manager, Infection Control & Tissue Viability, North Devon Healthcare NHS Trust. For responding to my last minute questions and sending me reading material I thank Professor Peter Molan of the Honey Research Unit, Waikato University, New Zealand. Thanks also to Stephen Pothecary of Comvita Ltd for clearing up some queries relating to manuka products. And thanks to the marketing department at Advancis Ltd for generously supplying me with samples of their manuka wound care products.

For a non-medical, non-scientific person such as me, the research and writing of this book has been quite a challenge. Always aware that I was 'punching above my weight' I have needed to take my time and plough through the facts, figures and research surrounding MRSA. Keeping a cool head and taking one day at a time, has been key to my ability as a researcher/author to write a factual and readable book. So my final thanks and gratitude go to Prem Rawat whose words of wisdom and gift of Knowledge have enabled me to find an inner strength and calm, even in the midst of the most stressful and difficult of days.

Introduction

Aromatherapy vs MRSA focuses solely on scientifically proven, antibacterial essential oils and their usefulness in the management of MRSA. Utilisation of essential oils for their therapeutic value was named 'aromatherapy' almost a hundred years ago. For more than thirty of those years I have worked with dozens of powerful and effective essential oils and consequently have not needed to consult a doctor since 1995. I have not taken an antibiotic since 1980 and so it was with incredulity, back in 2003, that I read an internet article about patients dying in hospital wards after becoming infected with the common bacterium *Staphylococcus aureus*. Having many years experience of essential oils clearing up nasty bacterial infections, I felt sure that MRSA would be no different - and my research began.

The first time I joined a meeting of the MRSA Support Group I thought I was at a meeting for ex-servicemen and women. There were amputees in wheelchairs, people using walking sticks and crutches – all victims of MRSA. Each disabled person was a civilian who had been in regular employment: the marketing man, now with a leg amputated above the knee; the accountant who could only walk with the aid of elbow crutches after MRSA had entered and destroyed a section of the long bones of his legs; the secretary whose abdominal wound refused to heal and was therefore unable to return to work. Each person had been relatively healthy when they entered hospital for a hip replacement, the routine setting of a broken bone, or removal of an appendix. Their battle had been fough in a hospital bed after MRSA bacteria had entered their body during, or shortly after, surgery.

The human immune system will do its best to protect the body from bacterial invasion and is primed to attack and fight microorganisms. Problems arise when antibiotics are given but don't work, then another antibiotic is tried and still may not work, but all the while the bacteria continue to multiply. Essential oils do not take the place of antibiotics as they cannot be given systemically, but by killing bacteria in a wound they can prevent a build up of bacteria. Unless the growth of bacteria is halted it progresses from contamination to colonisation, then to critical colonisation. When it eventually reaches a critical mass, it overwhelms the body's defence mechanisms, getting into the bloodstream and causing the serious condition, bacteraemia. Essential oils could also prove useful for pre-operative patients. If found to be MRSA positive, the patient is sent home with an antimicrobial body wash to replace normal household soap along with a pot of antibiotic cream to apply inside the nostrils. Patients are told, in no uncertain terms, that they have to decolonise or lose the position in the queue for surgery. Diluted essential oils can be used to cleanse and decolonise the body sites that are routinely swabbed during pre-surgery assessments, giving the patient 'a head start' when routinely used prior to an assessment.

MRSA is just a *Staphylococcus aureus*. This common bacterium, which we all carry as part of the normal flora of the body, is generally not harmful to humans. Some bacteria are pathogens, such as the ones that cause tuberculosis or meningitis. *Staph aureus* is one of the 'good' bacteria that live harmoniously on the skin, keeping pathogenic bacteria at bay. The problem we face is that *Staph aureus* has mutated to outwit the action of antibiotics and in so doing has become a 'superbug'. Because it can protect itself from being killed, it has been able to reproduce itself unchecked, and it is this multiplication factor of 'good' bacteria that makes it become 'bad'. To give an analogy, pure, clean water is not considered a dangerous substance. We are composed of 70% water; we would die if we were deprived of drinking water; we bathe in water; we cook with water. It only becomes a danger when there is too much of it; when it enters the lungs and death occurs. A small amount of *Staph aureus* is not a problem but controlling its growth in a patient's wound is critically important, as bacteria can double in number every twenty four hours, and so 1,000 bacteria on day one becomes 2,000 bacteria by day two, 4,000 bacteria by day 3, 64,000 on day 7, and by day 14 the bacterial count could have reached 8 million. But MRSA is not only confined to post-operative wounds, with many strains of MRSA now established in the community. Sadly, in the few years that community-associated MRSA has been affecting people many doctors have failed to diagnose the problem, as this new phenomenon was not previously part of medical school instruction. Training for doctors, in how to recognise the signs of MRSA, has recently been implemented, with guidelines being updated every time the bacteria mutates and changes its mode of attack.

Blame for MRSA infection is being apportioned to the government of the day or the cleanliness of a hospital, and although there may be culpability in each case, the main problem lies with the bacteria. Through the process of 'survival of the fittest' evolution has become the main culprit, although mankind has inadvertently helped the bacteria to mutate: self-medication being one of the many mistakes perpetuated. In some developing areas of the world, including India, Africa, and South America, a person can walk into a pharmacy and choose which antibiotic to purchase. A recent survey of 500 people in one African country showed that four out of five people self-medicated, and only went to a doctor for a diagnosis after repeated antibiotics had not worked. According to scientific reports another cause of multi-drug resistant *Staphylococcus aureus*, is 'bad decision making': from the feeding of antibiotics to agricultural animals as a prophylactic to keep them disease-free when they are forced to live in cramped, unsanitary conditions, to the over-prescribing of antibiotics by doctors because it hastens the patient from the surgery, and the folly in prescribing the same antibiotics for humans and animals. These and other reasons for antibiotic resistance are identified in Part Three, along with details of the organisations set up to deal with these important issues.

I have a great interest in the causes of disease, possibly because I grew up with an awareness of infection. My maternal grandmother died of post-operative septicaemia when I was a toddler, so I never knew her other than through photographs and stories related to me by my mother. My grandmother did not die from MRSA, as methicillin had not been introduced, but penicillin had failed to save her from a hospital-acquired infection. My mother had many operations in her lifetime and was proud of her scars. A scar is the outward, visible sign that a deep cut to the skin has healed. But after one operation, I remember my mother's wound did not heal, remaining open and messy for many weeks. Eventually she was readmitted to hospital for surgery to remove a surgical swab that had been accidentally left inside her. It is the body's natural urge to heal, by joining together the two edges of a wound and growing new skin. When a wound does not heal within a few weeks of surgery, the indications are that something is preventing healing from taking place.

Today there are untold numbers of people with wounds that will not heal. Many have been treated for an MRSA blood stream infection, and when no longer critically ill they are sent home. These patients are not being kept in hospital until they are cured. In UK hospitals there is a chronic shortage of beds and the only antibiotics that are powerful enough to tackle MRSA are so toxic that they can only be given, intravenously, for a short period of time. Even when the patient's life has been saved the infection is not always eradicated but there are no more effective antibiotics to take care of the residual MRSA. So patients are simply returned home and told to cope with the situation as best they can. Currently, there is no system for documenting how many people with MRSA-infected wounds are living in the community. What complicates matters even further is that post-operative patients are being sent home after three days, and it can take four, five or six days for an infection to manifest itself. Hospitals are places we have to go to, but by their very nature can be breeding grounds for MRSA. We need to do everything we can to protect ourselves and I have written this book as much a practical self-help guide, as a reference book on a serious subject. *Aromatherapy vs MRSA* is organised into three parts, allowing readers to access information of interest to them. Although structured, there is no running order and readers can dip into whichever section appeals. Each chapter stands alone, as do each of the appendices, and the book is designed more for reference than light reading.

Part One considers the unfolding story of MRSA, and its incredible ability to outwit antibiotics, and since microbiology testing has been crucial to our current knowledge of the antibacterial properties of essential oils, I invited a professor of microbiology to write a brief introduction to the processes used. There are two chapters contributed by academic experts in their field, and they are included for readers with an appetite to know more. Also in Part One is a snapshot of the international reach and zoonotic status of the superbug, with MRSA being documented in six out of the seven continents of the world. The superbug is affecting pets, horses and agricultural animals in several countries and has been detected on the meat we consume. A compilation of accounts of people damaged or killed by MRSA (both community and hospital-associated) has been added in order to illustrate the ferocity and diversity of MRSA infections. In the context of this book, each story may shock and move the reader to tears – as I was moved – but to the victims and their families, each account is a personal and ongoing tragedy. To everyone involved I offer my sympathy, along with my apologies for the impersonal nature of each tale, but I felt it was important to document a selection of MRSA-related injuries and deaths. The situation in North America is markedly different from that in Europe, with the majority of Europeans having little understanding of how terrifying MRSA can be.

Part Two focuses on the individual essential oils that have been scientifically proven to kill MRSA in laboratory settings. Research papers describe the antimicrobial action of essential oils: some inhibiting the growth of bacteria (bacteriostatic) and others with the ability to kill bacteria (bactericidal). Scientists in one university or hospital may use different protocols from scientists in another institution, so I have not attempted to compare results. One of the factors that makes a difference to the outcome is the amount of bacteria (the log) used at the beginning of each microbiology test, but very few papers give details of the log concentration. Another factor is the chemistry of the essential oil under test, as the specific ratio of aroma-chemicals that occur naturally in the plant can make a difference to its antibacterial activity. This may explain why researchers working independently of each other, can arrive at opposing conclusions, even though they are using the same essential oil and the same bacteria. Manuka honey is also documented in this section of the book, as there is evidence of a strong link between the essential oil chemistry in the manuka plant, and the potency of the honey. Every published paper is written in scientific language which can be extremely difficult to understand, so in order to keep the book as 'readable' as possible I have, on occasion taken the liberty of hyphenating some scientific terms in order to make the chapters a little easier for the non-scientist. Each paper has been condensed to a paragraph or two and readers can choose whether or not to access reference details at the end of the book.

Part Three is composed of a series of appendices: some to provide background information of general interest such as the time it took for *Staphylococcus aureus* to build resistance to each newly developed antibiotic, the length of time for MRSA to disseminate across Europe, the reasons for antibiotic resistance, and the risk factors involved. Some of the appendices offer practical guidance on how to use antimicrobial essential oils, and for people wishing to take an active role in their recovery I have included a section on the hygienic care of wounds. Preventative guidelines to on how people can protect themselves before, during and after, a hospital stay - implementation of these suggestions could help reduce the numbers of people developing MRSA - form another appendix. A resource section has been included as a practical self-help index for people who are booked for a pre-operative assessment, for those quietly suffering from chronic MRSA or those who have been damaged or bereaved by MRSA. The book concludes with a glossary to explain unfamiliar words or phrases.

My research began seven years ago when I contacted commercial microbiology laboratories in order to set up trials with essential oils and MRSA bacteria. Initial results inspired me to recruit volunteers from an MRSA support group and after encouraging feedback from using a blend of essential oils on their chronic wounds, I continued my research by working with microbiologists in the University of Brighton. A significant result with one essential oil was the spur that led me to write this book. Throughout, I have tried to give a fair representation of the MRSA problem, but it is by no means conclusive. New facts are uncovered on a regular basis as scientists identify and analyse the latest mutation. Ongoing research will undoubtedly add to existing information, but what is unquestionable is that mankind has become totally reliant on antibiotics: drugs that have only been developed, tested and marketed for the past seventy years. Within the timeframe of an average human lifespan we have come from celebrating the 'miracle of antibiotics' to a point where we now face a diminishing antibiotic effectiveness, when even minor surgery can be dangerous.

Yet there were effective antimicrobial products in general use long before antibiotics became the physicians' favourite medicine. Many natural products are capable of halting the growth of bacteria, and essential oils and blends of essential oils have a major part to play, along with garlic, silver, manuka honey and phage therapy - each the subject of extensive laboratory research with MRSA bacteria - all proven to be bacteriostatic, bactericidal or both. Antibiotics are losing the fight against MRSA and other superbugs, with leading scientists predicting that unless a solution is found soon, then 'we will be entering a pre-antibiotic era'. This statement could lead to fear and trepidation, but it fills me with optimism, because we now have, alongside empirical knowledge, the supporting scientific data that explains why and how natural remedies worked, killing bacteria and keeping people healthy long before the advent of penicillin.

Throughout *Aromatherapy vs MRSA*, I have brought together a mix of today's science with yesterday's 'tried and tested' remedies; from my recent research with combining different thyme oils to a create a potent blend, to the ancient knowledge that silver was a powerful germ killer. Within these pages you will find a great deal of interesting and helpful facts that may be useful – today, tomorrow or sometime in the future.

Part One
MRSA

A look at where we are and how we got here from the first
resistance developed by *Staphlococcus aureus*, to the sophistication
and adaption it shows to antibiotics today.

Chapter 1

MRSA – World View

MRSA is an international problem that affects the health of young and old alike. It can be picked up in the community as well as in hospitals and nursing homes. It is affecting the health of both domestic and agricultural animals. It has become adept at surviving long journeys. It can lie dormant on clothing and commercial items. It can be carried in the nostrils and on the bodies of healthy individuals. Researchers tracking the spread of MRSA say that the disease is distributed by the movement of people and goods around the world.

This chapter will look briefly at the MRSA research taking place in all corners of the globe. In particlar it will look at the burgeoning problem in the USA, which seems to be bearing the brunt of the newly emerging strains of the bacteria. Data gathering and infection monitoring is happening around the world. Fresh information constantly enters the public domain. This chapter is but a 'snapshot' of the problem of antibiotic resistance.

Countries with high antibiotic use also have a high MRSA rate. China and the USA are major consumers of antibiotics – China from both its sheer numbers and because it is now embracing Western medicine, the USA because of its large population with many uninsured, poor people often forced to purchase the cheapest available antibiotic from unregulated internet 'pharmacy' sites. Antibiotics are also freely available just over the border in Mexico, where there are streets lined with pharmacies selling every kind of prescription drug without need of a prescription. The North American antibiotic problem is compounded by the fact that farmers are feeding their agricultural animals vast amounts of antibiotics as a prophylactic.

A former director-general[1] of the World Health Organisation (WHO) said: "Used wisely and widely, the drugs we have today can be used to prevent the infections of today and the antimicrobial-resistant catastrophies of tomorrow. However, if the world fails to mount a more serious effort to fight infectious diseases, antimicrobial resistance will increasingly threaten to send the world back to a pre-antibiotic age."

The World Health Organization published a report in 1982, warning that the spread of antibiotic resistant bacteria in hospitals would make the choice of antibiotic 'a gamble of worsening odds'. Following this report, WHO initiated a survey of hospitals in fourteen countries which concluded that 'hospital infection is a common and serious problem throughout the world'. The following pages contain research independent of WHO.

A look at the global impact of MRSA

Australia

In the 1950s, a strain of *Staph aureus* infected new born babies in Australia. It then spread across much of the world, causing serious skin infections, sepsis and pneumonia in young adults and children. It was resistant to penicillin but was eradicated by methicillin in the 1960s. In 2005, an article in New Scientist magazine[2] reported on the discovery, by an international team of scientisits, that a newly identified clone of community-associated MRSA (CA-MRSA), called Southwest Pacific clone, was closely related to this 1950s *Staph aureus* strain. They also found that both these strains were closely related to epidemic strain EMRSA-16 which is commonly found in UK hospitals. In addition, the Southwest Pacific clone had spread to Europe causing fatal pneumonia in France, Sweden and Latvia.

In 2008 scientists[3] issued a warning that a new strain of MRSA had been detected in Australia. They named it the Queensland Clone, a deadly strain of MRSA that kills 50% of those it infects. It attacks lung tissue, leading to severe pneumonia. It is affecting teenagers and young adults who are otherwise healthy. When the bacteria gets into open wounds it destroys the layers between skin and muscle, preventing wounds from healing, and even a minor break in the skin can lead to severe boils. The Queensland Clone is resistant to antibiotics, whether singly or in combination. The principal scientist at Royal Perth Hospital said "MRSA is one of the biggest bacterial threats to humanity." The Queensland Clone, which is a CA-MRSA, is now being identified in the UK in people who have recently returned from Australia.

New Zealand

The incidence of MRSA in New Zealand is seen as low when compared to neighbouring Australia. In 1992, infectious control research[4] revealed that in the Auckland region there were a number of MRSA isolates with an unusual and distinctive pattern. Most of the people infected with this MRSA strain had recently arrived or returned from Western Samoa. The strain was named (WSPP) MRSA and was almost exclusively a CA-MRSA. It affected younger age groups, its virulence related to its toxin (PVL) production. The UK-derived EMRSA-15 was first recorded in 1998 and from that time onwards the WSSP-MRSA and the EMRSA-15 strains have jointly been dominant in New Zealand.

Japan

A Tokyo university microbiologist[5] was, in 1997, the first scientist to publish a paper on multi-drug (including vancomycin) resistance to bacteria, stating that 1967 was the 'golden age' of antibiotics. In 2004, a paper was published[6] discussing the progress of vancomycin resistance to MRSA, from its first detection in 1997 to the emergence of MRSA in other countries. Whereas some countries have a very low MRSA rate in hospitals, Japanese data[7] shows that MRSA accounts for 70% of all its hospital acquired infections, yet "no mechanism to identify patients with MRSA within hospitals currently exists in Japan." Reasons for the high proportion of MRSA rates in Japan are said to be related to the fact that antibiotic use is influenced by a pharmaceutical reimbursement system which provides incentives for physicians to prescribe them. This, combined with a low purchase price, encourages overuse. Because Japan has a generally healthy population with citizens living well into their 80s and 90s, the patients admitted to hospital are more likely to be the old and vulnerable; exceptional longevity may be a factor in the high incidence of MRSA in hospitals.

China

A study[8] carried out between 1999 and 2001, of all notified MRSA infections throughout China, Kuwait and the United States, showed that China had the highest level of MRSA resistance. Kuwait was the country with the second largest incidence of MRSA resistance. The USA came third. China was also shown to have the highest incidence of MRSA in its hospitals, accounting for 90% of all its hospital associated infections.

Korea

In 2007, research[9] carried out on CA and HA strains in Korea concluded that both were different from MRSA strains in other countries. Reports of a high prevalence of MRSA in Korea were reported[10] in 2000, after a man died from MRSA even though he had been treated with vancomycin and teicoplanin. A healthy young woman[11] who contracted CA-MRSA had to be hospitalised for more than 100 days. She survived, but required 6 weeks of vancomycin plus weeks of gentamicin. Two of her family members were found to test positive to MRSA, although not ill.

Kuwait

Researchers[12] from a Kuwait university conducted research with 26 community-associated MRSA strains. The results showed that two internationally recognized CA-MRSA clones were prevalent in Kuwait hospitals, and that these strains out-numbered HA-MRSA.

Turkey

In 2008, research in an Ankara hospital[13] screened 900 patients for MRSA on admission. Of the 900, eleven were found to have MRSA but only eight of the eleven had been hospitalized in the previous 12 months. Therefore it was surmised that only eight could have picked up an infection whilst an inpatient and that the other three had contracted MRSA in the community.

Russia

The first study[14] into the prevalence of MRSA in Russian hospitals showed that of all the *Staph aureus* clinical strains tested, just over one third were methicillin-resistant. MRSA rates varied significantly between hospitals and between wards, and there was no correlation between MRSA detection and geographical location of the hospital. The highest incidence of MRSA was in burns units at 78.4%, followed by ICUs with 41.3%, traumatic/orthopaedic surgery units 41.6% and lastly in general medical/surgical units 11.1%. In some hospitals the MRSA infection rate was 89.5% of all *Staph aureus* infections.

South Africa

A limited amount of researched and recorded data is available concerning South African MRSA infection rates. The following is taken from several sources. A study conducted across thirteen health-care institutions in just one province showed that antibiotic resistant *Staph aureus* was present in eleven of the facilities. The authors of the study[15] concluded that 'adequate infection control measures are urgently needed.' In 2004, an article in The Star newspaper[16] questioned whether the incidence of MRSA (known as Mister South Africa) which kills many people in South African hospitals, was being recorded as deaths from AIDS/HIV – "Aids patients dying from MRSA are almost certainly recorded as deaths from HIV". Furthermore, an orthopaedic surgeon[17] with expertise in osteomylitis (inflammation in the bone) said he comes across an average of twenty MRSA infections every month. He estimates that 80% of the *Staph aureus* in hospitals is MRSA. According to one of the country's top critical care specialists[18] the incidence of the superbug MRSA had, between 2000 and 2005, increased threefold.

Tanzania

A study was conducted in a medical centre to determine the prevalence of MRSA in the *Staph aureus* samples taken from patients in the facility. Results conclude that MRSA accounted for 16% of all *Staph aureus* isolates. This study[19] was triggered by a desire to compare Tanzanian MRSA rates with other African countries. "The prevalence of MRSA in eight countries from 1996 to 1997, was reported to be a relatively high 21% to 30% in Nigeria, Kenya and Cameroon, and relatively low, 10%, in Tunisia and Algeria".

India

Research carried out in Central India[20] into the prevalence of MRSA strains found that out of 280 *Staph aureus* strains studied, 51.8% were MRSA but all were susceptible to vancomycin. Research[21] in Chennai, South India found that 31% of *Staph aureus* isolates were MRSA. Throughout 2002, research in Northern India[22] found that methicillin resistance in *Staph aureus* was 38.56%. In 1999, a project showed that MRSA prevalence was 80.83% in a research centre[23]. This figure was compared with data taken from an earlier research project in the same establishment, which showed that the MRSA rate was just 12% in 1992.

Other research undertaken in India[24] into the speed at which bacteria have developed resistance to all but a few classes of antibiotics has so shocked scientists in the research hospital that they have implemented a regime of 'Strict Infection Control' in order to limit the indiscriminate use of antibiotics in situations such as surgical prophylaxis. However, the biggest problem is that throughout India, antibiotics can easily be purchased in any town or village pharmacy without a doctor's prescription, or even a diagnosis of the health condition.

Holland

The Netherlands has the lowest incidence of MRSA infection in the whole of Europe. In 2007,[25] the figure was 0.6%. The reasons are many. Firstly, from 1946, when antibiotics were made available, the Dutch authorities restricted their use to prescription only. The Dutch were able to monitor the emergence of MRSA across Europe and Scandinavia because the superbug took twenty-five years to reach Holland. They were adequately prepared and able to conduct a 'search and destroy' policy for every new admission to hospital. Health care workers are regularly screened for colonisation. If found to be positive, they are sent on sick leave until they test negative for MRSA. The small amount of MRSA found in the Netherlands is confined to hospitals, with no cases of CA-MRSA. Dutch belief is that "MRSA will never be solved by the introduction of new antibiotics."[26]

Sweden

The incidence of MRSA in Sweden has remained low since MRSA began spreading across Europe and Scandinavia. To see where the infection was originating from, a study[27] was set up to look at the number of cases imported into the country by travellers. Of the MRSA cases studied, over 75% were Swedish residents who had travelled or lived abroad and returned with an infection. The remainder of cases were made up from internationally adopted children, or immigrants and tourists to Sweden. Of all the imported MRSA cases, 55.4% were Hospital Associated and 32.9% were Community Associated. The majority of travellers had visited one or more of Thailand, United Kingdom, Greece, the former Yugoslavia, Lebanon, USA, Cyprus, Spain, Turkey or Syria.

Spain

During the period of 2004 to 2007, microbiologists in a Madrid hospital[28] collected thirteen PVL-positive MRSA isolates from patients attending the emergency department. Of the thirteen isolates, nine were from children, four from adults and all were associated with soft tissue infections. Nine of the thirteen had recently arrived from South America, demonstrating the trans-continental movement of CA-MRSA. In Brazil and other countries in South America, antibiotics are easily obtainable without a prescription, and consequently there is very high antibitoic resistance.

Iceland

Since 1991, Icelandic hospital authorities have implemented a 'search and destroy' policy to screen and identify patients for the presence of MRSA. Patients with identified risk factors were screened; the objective was to identify and decolonise carriers in order to keep hospitals free of MRSA. The incidence of MRSA is low, but rising, in comparison to most other European countries. Microbiological data and clinical samples collected between the years 2000 – 2008, were retrospectively analysed[29] in order to gain understanding of why the incidence of MRSA was growing despite the stringent hospital policies. Analysis showed that from 2000 to 2003, two HA-MRSA strains were dominant, and that both had been successfully contained with infection control measures. After 2004, there was seen to be a growing number of CA-MRSA infections in people with no relation to the health care system. Of the variety of MRSA strains identified, it was found that the USA300 and the Southwest Pacific (SWP) strains were most common, reflecting an influx of MRSA from other countries. A significant proportion of the isolates were PVL positive. Although the incidence of MRSA in Iceland has increased since 1999, it has remained low owing to the effective screening measures in place. The research paper concluded that "MRSA in Iceland is now shifting into the community, challenging the current Icelandic guidelines, which are tailored to the health care system."

United Kingdom

MRSA was first seen in the UK in 1961. Fifty years later, although the problem of MRSA infection is never far from the headlines, the exact number of people affected by MRSA is unknown. The voluntary surveillance of *Staph aureus* bacteraemias which began in 1989, became mandatory in 2001. This showed that the proportion of *Staph aureus* infections that were antibiotic resistant increased from 2% in 1990, to around 40% in in the early 2000s. There is a relationship between the rise in bacteraemia infections and the emergence of epidemic strains EMRSA-15 and EMRSA-16. The Health Protection Agency (HPA) records all HA-MRSA infection deaths and states the most recent figures to be under 2,000 a year, down from the oft quoted figure of 5,000 a year. These figures refer only to people whose blood tests show the presence of MRSA in the bloodstream (bacteraemia) at the time of death. There are no figures to reflect the number of people who have survived an MRSA infection and been discharged from hospital but who are still unwell as a result.

Hospital Associated MRSA is still the dominent type within the UK although CA-MRSA (PVL) has increased ten fold in the years between 2005 - 2010. In preparation for an upsurge in cases, the Health Protection Agency has in place a PVL management recomendation[30] on its website. The head of the Staphylococcus Reference Unit (SRU)[31] said, in February 2011: "Confirming that PVL is the cause of the majority of staphylococcal boils and abscesses referred to the HPA in England is a significant step in our understanding of this infection and has helped to improve treatment for patients presenting to their GPs with these conditions. GPs now have immediate access to the guidelines on the HPA's website which give a succinct step-by-step guide to the most appropriate treatment for boils and abscesses caused by PVL infection."

There is no data to quantify the numbers of people who have had amputations as a result of contracting MRSA, nor data to show how many people have been crippled in other ways by MRSA. The true number of MRSA-affected people in the UK is estimated by experts to be in the hundreds of thousands.

Carriage of MRSA is another important subject. One UK professor[32] says: "The carrier state is an absolute menace, because if you have carrier patients they have to be isolated from other patients. If you have a surgeon who is a carrier you have to stop him operating, and that is extremely difficult." Pre-admission swabbing of patients for elective surgery alerts hospitals as to which people are already colonised, so that they are not admitted to hospital, and therefore cannot infect their own surgical sites nor infect other patients. Anyone testing positive for MRSA is given chlorhexedine and mupirocin to take home and told to 'get themselves clear', otherwise they can not have their elective operation. However, no such precautions can be taken for emergency surgery.

USA

In the US, the highest rates of hospital associated infections are found in patients in ICUs, followed by patients in other hospital departments, then in out-patient departments. The US Centers for Disease Control (CDC) recorded a 36% rate of *Staph aureus* infections in ICUs in 1992. By 2003, the MRSA rate was 65% of the total of ICU infections.

A 1977 survey[33] estimated that every year in the United States, somewhere between 70,000 – 140,000 new cases of antibiotic resistant infection resulted in approximately 18,000 deaths (not only MRSA). A study[34] in 1994, estimated that the death rate from infections, mostly involving drug resistant bacteria, were 65,000 – 70,000 a year. A research company[35], in its marketing material, stated in 2007, "we have 2 million infections a year from MRSA with 80,000 – 90,000 deaths."

The CDC estimated that between 1999 and 2000, more than 125,000 people a year were hospitalised for MRSA infections. People living in the southern part of the US were more likely to be affected, as the hot and humid environment is an ideal breeding ground for bacteria. In 2001, a San Francisco hospital ER department was treating so many MRSA-CA boils and abscesses that it had to open a special clinic for skin infections.

A new community MRSA strain was identified in 2000, and named USA 300. By 2009, it had become the most prevalent MRSA strain in many hospitals. In 2006, the USA 300 (extra-virulent) strain was identified. This strain is resistant to many more antibiotics than earlier CA-MRSA strains, including mupirocin, which has been widely relied upon for topical treatment and decolonisation of patients. CA-MRSA now accounts for 70% of all reported MRSA infections in some parts of the USA.

Recent data from the CDC show that during the US flu season of 2007-2008, there were seventy-four child deaths from influenza and that twenty two of the children were also infected with MRSA. The CDC is now implementing a monitoring network for patients co-infected with flu and MRSA during flu seasons, in order to prevent flu-MRSA cases from resulting in fatalities.

In conclusion, according to a 2005 report by the United States Centers for Disease Control, Community Associated MRSA was responsible for

94,000 life-threatening infections resulting in around 19,000 deaths in the USA. Little or no published information is available on the health status of the 75,000 survivors, although there are several websites where survivors of MRSA can talk to other sufferers. In comparison to the epidemic of CA-MRSA in the USA, the incidence of CA-MRSA in the UK is relatively small but had, between 2005 to 2010, increased ten fold.

Summary

Although the above examples are only a snapshot of MRSA infection around the world, it is clear that mankind's most common bacterial adversary is not only gaining in virulence and invincibility, but also increasing in the speed at which it can destroy a human life. It has joined 'the jet set', travelling between continents as easily and quickly as humans, livestock, cargo and baggage.

Chapter 2
MRSA – Human Stories

MRSA used to be considered a healthcare-associated disease that only affected patients with established risk factors such as the hospitalised elderly or children and babies with serious ailments. In both instances the vulnerability would stem from a weakened immune system. A form of MRSA has emerged in the community which is known as community associated MRSA (CA-MRSA) as it affects people with no interaction with a health care facility and who don't necessarily fall into one of the lifestyle risk factors for CA-MRSA, such as intravenous drug use. The term CA-MRSA, coined in 2000, is microbiologically distinct from hospital associated MRSA (HA-MRSA) and is treated with a different selection of antibiotics. What differentiated the two was that HA-MRSA was harder to treat as only a small selection of antibiotics are effective. CA-MRSA was generally considered easier to treat as a wider range of antibiotics could successfully be used. The problem is that CA-MRSA is very fast acting and, if it affects the lungs, can kill an otherwise healthy individual within 24 hours of diagnosis. Reports of sudden death from CA-MRSA were being published on the website of the US Centers for Disease Control and Prevention (CDC) until recently. Throughout North America, doctors are being trained in what to look for and being made aware of the necessity of speedy and correct action in order to minimise adverse outcomes.

The following stories are of both HA-MRSA and CA-MRSA infections. The people affected are from both the United Kingdom and the United States. Some survived an infection of MRSA and sadly, others did not. Their stories are all unique. What binds them together is *Staphylococcus aureus*. This common bacterium, has now evolved to a point where it has out-smarted many antibiotics, and is continuing to evolve in order to survive the ones that are still useful. The current antibiotic routinely used to treat HA-MRSA is vancomycin, which can only be given intravenously and only for a short period of time. It is very toxic, with side effects that include kidney damage. Antibiotics such as daptomycin, prescribed for the treatment of boils and cellulitis caused by CA–MRSA, can clear up the MRSA infection temporarily, only for it to return. The bacteria can be diminished but not entirely eradicated from the body and, like a battalion of soldiers that has retreated for strategic reasons, regroups and fights again.

These stories are just a handful amongst thousands. MRSA causes loss of life, and as deeply tragic as this is, it is unfortunately but the tip of the iceberg. Many more people have lost limbs, fingers or toes, normal mobility, their energy, their memory, or the freedom to leave their house because of constantly discharging wounds. Some are denied the option of living a healthy life without regular visits to hospital for operations to have bacteria physically scraped from inside their body. Many more suffer terrible depression as their chronic state of ill health forces radical changes to their lives.

Loss of a leg

In the year 2000, Mr. F. from Yorkshire was a fit and healthy marketing man in his late 40s, who one day lost his balance, fell down a flight of stairs, and broke his leg. It was a vertical break that went into the knee joint. His leg became very swollen, and surgery was undertaken before the swelling had gone down. Within days of the operation he felt very unwell. Blood tests showed that he had a serious infection for which he was prescribed an antibiotic called linezolid, and the wound was closed. He was barrier nursed for the next eight weeks and then discharged from hospital. Just one week later he felt very ill. His family took him to the Accident & Emergency department of his local hospital where x-rays were taken. The x-ray plates showed black holes in his leg that indicated an abscess from his thigh to his ankle. He needed emergency surgery to remove the abscessed material. His leg was saved with the use of bone paste and plastic surgery, taking muscle from his back. He was then put into a hot room with a constant 80° temperature for two months. When he was eventually sent home one leg was shorter than the other and he had to learn to walk with crutches. In 2003, he developed cellulitis in the leg. He was told that MRSA was still in the bone and that he had to decide between two fates: either to have his leg amputated above the knee or to spend a week in hospital, four times a year, for the rest of his life. As he had already suffered so much discomfort and distress from the medical procedures over the previous two years, he opted for amputation. It was a further 18 months before he was completely clear of MRSA, and it was Spring 2005, before his leg was healed. Because the amputation was above the knee he found it too painful to walk with prosthetic devices and relies on a wheelchair for his mobility.

Nancy's story

Nancy is a woman in her 60s living in Florida. In January 2006, she was fit and healthy. During a visit to her daughter in Ohio her hands began to swell. She went to the Emergency Room of the local hospital where she was given steroid injections, but she became more ill over the next few days. Tests eventually confirmed a diagnosis of MRSA. She was given intravenous antibiotics and moved to a bigger hospital when MRSA was found in her pericardium as well as her bloodstream. The intravenous vancomycin had to be stopped when her kidneys began to fail and her family thought she was going to die. It took forty five days of treatment before she was well enough to go home with a PICC line and further antibiotics. For the next two years she had to take antibiotics on a continuous basis. She was told the MRSA was 'dormant' in her body and could flare up again. A full four years since the initial illness, she is still taking low dose antibiotics as a 'just in case' scenario.

A broken wrist

In 2004, a 31 year old British woman slipped whilst on the deck of a boat, breaking her wrist. In the Accident and Emergency department of the nearest hospital pins were inserted into her wrist to help the break heal correctly, and she was sent home. Three days later she noticed bleeding through the cast. She returned to the hopsital to report the problem and was told not to worry, and sent home. Ten days later she had a fever, was in intense pain and aware of a bad smell coming from inside the cast. Again she returned to the hospital. This time the cast was removed to reveal the wound as green and purulent. Swabs taken confirmed MRSA. An operation was required to clean out the wound, after which she was sent home with a course of antibiotics. Instead of halting the growth of bacteria, the antibiotics failed to work and the bacteria started to eat through her skin. Eventually she was given an antibiotic that did work and the infection cleared up, but she is left with an inch-long scar and a permanently weakened wrist.

Knee replacement

In 2003, a 71 year old American woman went into hospital for elective surgery. She needed to have a knee replacement, which is usually a straightforward procedure. Whilst in hospital she developed septic shock due to an infection in her upper leg and was treated with the powerful antiboiotic vancomycin. Antibiotic therapy led to an improvement in the symptoms but the MRSA was not killed and eventually her leg had to be amputated in order to save her life.

Pneumonia

During the mid-2000s, in the United States, a healthy 17 year old high school girl complained one day about a sore throat. She took time off school to recover but three days later she was taken to her doctor who diagnosed pneumonia, and she was admitted to hospital. An array of tests were completed. Two days later her parents were informed that their daughter had MRSA. They were assured that the antibiotics would soon clear it up, but over a period of four months the prescribed cocktail of antibiotics failed to work. After every effort by medical staff, using all available drugs, equipment and procedures, nothing was able to save her life.

A boil on the buttock

In 2005, a young mother in the United States developed a boil on her buttock. A doctor lanced the boil and prescribed an antibiotic. A few weeks later she returned to her doctor as there was an additional area of inflammation on her inner knee. She was given an intravenous antibiotic whilst in the doctor's office and sent home. The following day she felt no better and returned to her doctor, where swabs confirmed that she was infected with MRSA. A week later she was told that her infection was the very serious necrotising fasciitis, and that she would need to undergo emergency surgery in order to save her leg and possibly her life. High doses of vancomycin and emergency surgery were followed by daily wound care. Afterwards, further surgery was performed to graft new skin over the wound. She made a slow recovery over the next two months, developing blood clots from lack of mobility. She needed months of physical therapy to repair nerve damage, but luckily this woman survived CA-MRSA.

The sports-crazy

19 year old In 2003, in the United Kingdom, a 19 year old sports-crazy boy, who was physically fit and very healthy, took a tumble whilst training and landed badly on one knee. He was admitted to hospital for emergency repair to the dislocated knee, damaged ligaments and severed artery. Both the emergency and follow-up surgery were pronounced successful, but a few days later he began experiencing flu-like symptoms which were eventually confirmed as MRSA and he was re-hospitalised. For several weeks he was kept in an isolation room, on intravenous antibiotics, whilst all metal pins were removed from his knee. His eventual discharge from hospital came three months after the accident. Back at home, he was mostly bedbound and easily fatigued. Depression swiftly followed, as the young fit sportsman was unable to resume his previous lifestyle. Years later he is still experiencing pain. Although he has learnt to walk again, he has been told he might never be able to run.

A 12 year old with pneumonia

In 2007, a healthy and athletic boy of twelve from the United States went on a school camping trip. On his return he looked pale and was running a fever. A day later he was coughing and lethargic so his parents took him to hospital for assessment. He was diagnosed with pneumonia, given a course of antibiotics and sent home. Just one day later he became very ill and was rushed back to hospital. He was put into an induced coma and connected to a ventilating machine. Body fluid samples taken previously confirmed he was seriously ill with MRSA. Although all available antibiotics were given, over the next two weeks his organs shut down one by one and he was artifically kept alive. Eventually his parents acknowledged that their son would not recover and he was removed from the life support machines.

A 21 year old college student

In 2003, in the USA, a physically fit and strong 21 year old college football player consulted the family doctor when he had flu-like symptoms. The doctor was concerned that there was something more serious that needed investigating and had him admitted to hospital. The young man was given five different antibiotics and put on a ventilator, but when their treatment did not work the doctors were baffled. They did not know what was attacking the previoulsy healthy young man, and a few days later he died. An autopsy revealed that he had contracted MRSA from a pimple on his buttock.

An American football player

In the year 2000, an American football player in his early thirties went into hospital for a routine operation to his knee. After about a week at home he noticed a hot area above the operation site and was experiencing flulike symptoms. Two days later he was back in hospital and the infection had spread over a large area of his leg. He was taken into surgery so that the infection, newly confirmed as MRSA, could be washed out. He was then sent home with a PICC line for six weeks of intravenous vancomycin. The side effects of vancomycin included intense itchiness and reddening of the skin and he was subsequently switched to linezolid. Treatment seemed to be successful and he was given a clean bill of health. Several months later he suffered a second knee injury, which resulted in him experiencing similar symptoms as before. He was re-admitted to hospital for further surgery to again have the infection cleaned out. Months of antibiotic therapy followed, and he also needed treatment for bloodclots in his lungs. He survived the MRSA infection but became terrified of incurring further sports injuries in case this precipitated further MRSA infections.

Hip replacement surgery

In 2005, a man from the north of England, with terrible pains in his leg, was misdiagnosed and advised that he could still go on holiday. Pain increased during the holiday and the local hospital diagnosed a fractured hip, which led to an operation for a half-hip replacement. A week after the operation he was discharged from hospital even though he still had a weeping wound. Back in his home town he was re-admitted to hospital where, over the following weeks, the formerly strong and courageous man became weaker and weaker until he could no longer bear to eat food. His wife was helpless to do anything, and could only sit by her husband's bedside as his health deteriorated. MRSA had swept through his body in a period of eight weeks, destroying his kidneys, liver and lungs. Eventually, the hospital staff admitted that there was absolutely no chance of his recovery and announced that they would be switching off the life support machines. His death certificate stated: Pneumonia and MRSA Septacaemia plus organ failure.

A toddler

In the spring of 2004, an American boy, just past his first birthday, became very ill. His family doctor prescribed antibiotics and steroids. At first he seemed to recover but two weeks into the antibiotic treatment he awoke one morning with a high fever and in great distress. His parents took him to the Emergency Room of their nearest hospital, where doctors examined him and sent him home. Later that day he was rushed back to hospital when his breathing became laboured, and from the Emergency Room he was transferred to the Intensive Care Unit. His parents were informed that their son had gone into septic shock and that he was a very sick child. He died the following day. It was not until an autopsy was performed that the cause of death was acknowledged to be MRSA. A previously healthy child had been killed by toxins released by the bacteria which had attacked his organs, causing death within 24 hours of being admitted to hospital.

Author's notes

Each one of the above accounts has occurred since the year 2000: even though MRSA was seen as problematic in the 1990s, the CA-MRSA strains have become increasingly virulent since the mid 2000s. The main causes of MRSA fatality fall into a few broad categories.

Sometimes human error is involved: when a wound has been sewn up too soon, with bacteria trapped inside the body. As this is a case of medical negligence, in the UK it is the only cause of an MRSA infection that stands a good chance of winning a legal case.

Sometimes a death (that may have been averted had doctors recognised an MRSA infection in a timely manner) occurs even after robust attempts to save the life of the patient. Although this is also human error, it is, sadly, a common occurrence and very difficult to prove as medical negligence.

Sometimes the speed at which death occurred could not have been prevented. Initial symptoms mimicked those of the influenza virus, but instead of being able to 'sweat it out' as most people are able to do before recovering from a bout of flu, the MRSA bacteria has quickly entered the lungs, causing fatal pneumonia. The virulence factor of some CA-MRSA strains in the USA has become so fast acting and deadly in outcome that it could be likened to being bitten by a poisonous snake, for which there is no anti-venom serum.

Becoming infected with MRSA, in any of its forms, is a truly terrifying and dangerous event. As yet, there is no promise of a reprieve, and we wait for our governments to instigate the rigorous research necessary for the provision of adequate medical intervention. In the meantime, each one of us needs to be aware of this health threat, both in our hospitals and in our communities. We need to have an awareness of the signs and symptoms of MRSA infection and if recognising them in ourselves or in a family member, we need to make our voice heard. When something is seriously wrong with our body we are the ones who should know, who should not allow ourselves be sent home, but with respect and perseverance ask the medical personnel, "Are you absolutely sure this is not MRSA?" Some diseases 'run their course' and little intervention is required but this is not the situation with MRSA, where a speedy diagnosis with efficient treatment could make the difference between life and death.

In North America the number of MRSA deaths outnumber those from AIDS by a factor of five, yet current funding for MRSA research is just a tiny fraction of the funding available for HIV/AIDS research.

Chapter 3
MRSA in Animals

Animals do not catch chicken pox or measles from their human owners, nor do we catch feline influenza or distemper from our cats or dogs. In general, animal diseases are specific to animals and human diseases are specific to humans. Rarely does a disease cross the species barrier. When it does, it is called a zoonotic disease. MRSA has recently been classified as a zoonotic disease as it affects both humans and animals and can be transferred from one to the other.

There are dozens of species of *staphylococci*, but the three most important species to humans are *Staphylococcus aureus*, *Staphylococcus epidermidis* and *Staphylococcus saprophyticus*. *Staph aureus* is the only *staphylococcus* that affects both humans and animals. Our companion animals are affected by *Staph aureus*, *Staph intermedius* and *Staph psuedo-intermedius*, a sub-category of *Staph intermedius*. In dogs, it is *Staph intermedius* that is the main cause of cystitis and suppurative disease, such as the pus-filled ulcers known as pyodermic. In cats it causes skin tumours, boils and abcesses, known as pyogenic.

In Korea[1], where the human MRSA incidence is 50% of all *Staph aureus* infections, a study of MRSA infected animals suggested that once the disease crossed between human and animal, these isolates, or specific types of bacteria, would become prevalent throughout the veterinary world. "Resistance in bacteria isolated from food animals has been suspected as a potential source of resistance in human pathogens."

MRSA has been a cause for concern amongst humans for several decades and documented as a problem in agricultural animals since the 1970s. It was only recognized as a problem in the small animal veterinary world in the late 1990s, when an increasing number of infections in dogs, cats and other companion animals – horses in particular – were diagnosed.

The majority of pet owners are unaware that their animals could be susceptible to an infection that is sometimes life threatening. It is not widely understood that the use of antibiotics in agricultural animals, which end up as meals for both humans and pets, is compounding the threat of MRSA.

The situation is already worrying. There are voices of reason trying to educate government, medical personnel and the public about the correct use of antibiotics. In 1997, an alliance, RUMA[2] was formed to "promote the highest standards of food safety, animal health and human health as well as ensure minimal damage to the environment." Their mantra, on the use of antimicrobials, is "use as little as possible but as much as needed."

Cats and dogs

Companion animals, mainly cats and dogs, can act as a reservoir, or carrier, for MRSA. This was observed in a geriatric hospital ward where MRSA was prevalent amongst the patients. A ward cat was good company for the elderly patients and was considered to be helpful in their recovery, but the problem of MRSA became persistent. The ward staff were swabbed and found to be carriers of MRSA in their nostrils. The cat, also swabbed, was found to be heavily colonised with MRSA. After its removal, and in tandem with infection control measures, the MRSA rate amongst the geriatric patients began to decline. In 2005, a study of MRSA isolates from companion animals revealed that 93.5% were the same as MRSA isolates from epidemic MRSA commonly found in UK healthcare settings.

According to information gathered by the Royal Veterinary College[3] the early incidence of MRSA in companion animals was noted as follows:

1999	Eleven dogs in UK, USA, and Korea.
2003	One dog in the Netherlands.
	95 isolates of MRSA recorded at one UK laboratory.[4]
2004	Seven dogs and five cats in UK.
2005	Since this year there have been more than 50 papers written on MRSA in pets.

In 2009 an analysis of swabs taken, over a period of years, from MRSA infected cats and dogs in Europe were as follows:

- epidemic strain EMRSA-15   95.4%

- epidemic strain EMRSA-16   1.6%

- Other MRSA strain   3.0%

In 2004, in the UK, the first recorded death of a dog from the human form of MRSA spurred its owner to set up an educational foundation[5] in order to create awareness of the dangers of MRSA infections in veterinary clinics and hospitals. Within weeks of the website going live, emails were pouring in from pet owners, veterinary and human health practitioners, journalists, wildlife animal keepers and farmers, all wanting to know more about the risks of cross infection of MRSA between humans and animals. From 2005 to the present day, the ongoing educational campaign is resulting in improved hygiene of veterinary practices[6] and better barrier nursing of MRSA-infected pets in veterinary establishments on both sides of the Atlantic.

If your cat or dog has a wound that refuses to heal, and if you have recently been in hospital and have been treated for MRSA, then it is advisable to inform your vet so that they can have blood samples analysed to see if your pet's problem is MRSA colonising the wound, and preventing healing from taking place.

Conversely, if you have been treated for MRSA and have been sent home with a clean bill of health, but can't quite seem to regain full health, it is possible that your pet is a carrier of MRSA. Even though the pet doesn't seem to be affected by MRSA, every time you stroke him/her you may be unknowingly becoming reinfected. You need to tell your vet of your recent illness and say that you suspect your animal could be a carrier. Have some tests carried out, so that both you and your pet can be decolonised.

People with chronically infected wounds and/or colonised areas of the body, could potentially colonise their pets. A study conducted in the early 2000s, has shown that pets can become colonised and their wounds can become infected with MRSA when the owners are themselves affected. Both pet and owner need to be treated.

Cross infection between pet owners and pets is now a fact of life. If a wound is not healing up and you have a pet, it is advisable to take your animal to the vet for swabs to be taken. Your vet will then send the swabs to a diagnostic laboratory and if results show that your pet is carrying MRSA on its coat or in its nostrils, it is important to have the animal treated with antimicrobials so that you are not re-contaminated with MRSA.

Similarly, if you have a pet with a wound that is not healing up, and you work in a hospital, nursing home, or correctional facility, or are a visitor to a hospital, then you should consider having your self swabbed and diagnosed, as you may be carrying MRSA which is being transfered to your animal. In the UK, it may be difficult, if not impossible, to persuade your doctor to take a swab, as the UK healthcare services are underfunded and this diagnostic procedure would not be considered as critical. It may be necessary to contact a private laboratory[7] so that you can have swabs taken and analysed for your MRSA status. Although the cost is not insignificant, it may in the long run save you money on continuing veterinary fees.

Within the UK it is widely believed that CA-MRSA is not as yet, and will not become, a problem in companion animals, but in the USA, researchers have detected PVL toxin in twenty three animal isolates of MRSA.[8] They say: "this is the first study to demonstrate the presence of the PVL toxin genes in MRSA strains isolated from companion animals." The results are noteworthy in that MRSA strains that produce the PVL toxin have been shown in many studies to cause pneumonia, necrotizing dermatitis, and other primary diseases in humans and that these conditions were mirrored in animals. It would seem that the MRSA situation in the USA, in both humans and animals, is pointing towards CA-MRSA, with the addition of the PVL toxin in a significant number of cases. In the UK, the current status of MRSA, in both humans and animals is predominantly HA-MRSA.

Key points
- If you have an infected wound that won't clear up – suspect your dog or cat! Ask your vet to take swabs and send them off to a diagnostic laboratory. Your vet should get the results within a few days and then you will need to discuss the options available for decolonising your pet. Or, you can set up your own system for decolonising your pet. Either way you will also need to address the problem of your own colonisation and seek suitable treatment.

- If you have a pet whose wound will not clear up, suspect that you could be a carrier and have yourself checked out. I understand that UK doctors will often refuse this type of request as there is an expense involved, and each health care practice has a budget to manage. In the USA, where all medical procedures are paid for either by direct invoice or insurance, it would be straightforward to request that swabs be taken for analysis.

- At the moment, the MRSA strains infecting cats and dogs are predominantly EMRSA-15 and EMRSA-16, the same strains of MRSA causing problems in hospitals.

- CA-MRSA has not yet been detected in animals with an MRSA infection in the UK, but is being seen in the USA.

- Antimicrobial resistance in the veterinary world is increasing in the same way that it is increasing in the human population.

- Humans are more likely to acquire an MRSA infection if they have had several courses of antibiotics for recurrent infections, and the same is true for dogs and cats.

- Pet owners who work in a healthcare facility such as a clinic, hospital or nursing home, have a significantly higher chance of being an MRSA carrier than other pet owners.

- Veterinary staff could be MRSA carriers. Just as humans are being urged to ask their doctors and nurses, "have you washed your hands?" it is as important to see that the person handling your pet has done so or is wearing a pair of sterile gloves. Don't be embarrassed about asking. You have the right to expect the highest standards of care for your beloved pet, and you are paying for every visit.

- Whereas it is permissable for you to treat your own pet, it is illegal to treat someone else's pet unless you are a trained veterinarian.

Horses

Equine MRSA is thought to be disseminated internationally. Many studies[9] have taken place around the world to look into the extent of nasal colonisation, and if there is, whether it has any significant impact on human health. There is a question over the origin of MRSA in horses. It is not clear whether the source has been from human transmission or has entered the horse population from agricultural animals.

The possibility of humans being responsible for the transfer of MRSA to animals was considered back in 1999, when eleven horses were admitted to a veterinary hospital for various medical procedures. Over a thirteenmonth period, all eleven needed to return just two to three weeks after being discharged. All the horses were re-admitted with surgical wound infections, which when swabbed and analysed, confirmed they each had MRSA.

When five surgical staff were also swabbed, it was shown that three were colonised with MRSA, even though they were otherwise healthy. The conclusion was that the source of the MRSA outbreak was most probably of human origin as the horses had arrived at the hospital over an extended period of time and from several locations, yet none of the horses had presented with a *staph* infection on arrival.

Equine vets, in general, are confident that because horses spend much of their time outside in fresh air, even if they do become colonised with MRSA in their stables, then they can quickly decolonise once they are returned to the field.

• In the 1990s, Japanese researchers[10] conducted research with equine isolates of MRSA but failed to make a link with human isolates of MRSA. Similar research has also taken place in Canada and the UK, where equine strains of MRSA were found to be different from the most prevalent human strains in the UK: EMRSA-15 and EMRSA-16.

• Throughout Canada[11] the predominant clone affecting horses is Canadian MRSA-5, which is the same as USA500. This MRSA strain, which was human in origin, accounts for only a small percentage of infections in the human population but is common in horses.

• Some studies of MRSA colonisation in horses put the figure between 3% and 10% of healthy horses. Whilst uncommon among horses in general, MRSA can cluster on farms.[12] It is rare for a colonised horse to develop an MRSA infection, although it has been noted[13] that colonisation at the time of admission to an equine hospital was seen as a risk factor in the subsequent development of a clinical MRSA infection.

• When horses are colonised with MRSA, the most important factor in reducing the spread among other horses and equine personnel is good hygiene, which mirrors infection control measures in veterinary clinics and human hospitals.

Agricultural animals

Animals reared as meat products are all regularly treated with antibiotics in order to keep infections to a minimum, as farmed animals are generally kept in closer proximity to each other than would naturally occur if the animals had a choice in the matter. In addition to animals needing antibiotics to clear up problems such as mastitis in dairy cows, it was, until fairly recently, possible for individual farmers to purchase antibiotics as growth enhancers. It was not until 2002, that such unregulated use of antibiotics was recognized as a threat to human health. The European Union outlawed this practice in 2006, but in the United States the use of unprescribed antibiotics as growth promoters has continued unchecked. Some prominent researchers[14] led by Dr. Stuart Levy formed an organisation with the explicit intent of bringing about a conscious appraisal of antibiotic use in veterinary as well as human medicine. In July 2009, the US administration and FDA (Food & Drug Administration) called for the phasing out of antimicrobial drugs for growth promotion and feed efficiency. The new approach will also require that all useage of antibiotics must be carried out under the supervision of a veterinarian rather than as now, which is at the discretion of the farmer. This would see an end to over-the-counter sales of, literally, tons of antimicrobial drugs.

In veterinary medicine it has been shown that certain *staphylococcus* species are significant in specific diseases. *Staph aureus* causes mastitis in cattle, sheep, goats and horses, and dermatitis in sheep and goats. *Staph hyicus* causes arthritis in pigs. It is the overuse of antibiotics in agricultural animals that has contributed to the problem of MRSA in the animals themselves, and in the transference of MRSA from the animal carcasses to humans working in abattoirs and butchers. Ongoing research will determine exactly how critically the overuse of antibiotics in agricultural animals has contributed to the prevalence of MRSA in humans.

Over the past four decades much research has been carried out into the health of farmed animals, and some interesting results have been obtained.

- In 1975, it was reported[15] that MRSA was found in isolates of mastitis in twenty Belgian dairy herds. It was thought that the infection came from a single human source. MRSA can be transferred from human to cow and/or cow to man, if the MRSA bacteria has colonised milking machines. Dairy cows are prone to suffering from mastitis as their udders are now far larger than is normal and they are regularly prescribed antibiotics to clear up the infection.

• A 2006 survey in Holland uncovered the uncomfortable fact that 20% of pork products were infected with MRSA. A strain[16] of MRSA had infected factory-farmed pigs. The same strain was also detected in chicken and beef. As well as Holland, the MRSA strain was found in Denmark, Belgium, Germany and the United Kingdom. Although not widespread, the problem is still serious as MRSA can infect anyone who touches an infected animal: vet, farmer, abattoir worker, butcher and possibly also the end user – the person who cooks the meat. Although it is thought that MRSA is killed by cooking, a danger exists when the meat is still raw. Whilst the risk of MRSA reaching the meat we consume is relatively small, there is a need for correct cooking and good kitchen hygiene, as poorly cooked meat could allow colonisation of the human gut.

• When a Canadian veterinary college[17] tested a batch of uncooked pork chops for the presence of MRSA bacteria it was found in 10% of the samples.

• In the United States a group of epidemiologists[18] conducted studies on a large pig farm by taking and analysing swabs from the pigs' noses. It was found that 70% of the pigs were colonised with MRSA. Swine workers were found to be colonised when tested in a later research programme.[19]

• The Infectious Diseases Society of America (IDSA)[20] has stated: "Infectious disease physicians and public health advocates are greatly concerned about the growing body of scientific evidence demonstrating that antimicrobial drug use in livestock and poultry contributes to the spread of drug-resistant bacteria to people."

• A comprehensive study of MRSA in animals, covering companion animals, horses, and livestock, both poultry and mammals, has been published by The Soil Association.[21] It contains a vast amount of information on the emerging international problem of MRSA in domestic and agricultural animals: "organic farming methods are beneficial for the environment but they also reduce the need for antibiotics as young animals are allowed to stay with their mother until weaned. Farmed pigs, for example, are weaned early before their immune systems are mature and are therefore vulnerable to infections and consequently antibiotics are routinely added to the feed of farmed swine."

- The use of antibiotics in farmed animals differs greatly from country to country. The UK allows the prophylactic, or disease prevention, use of antibiotics in animal feed, whereas Holland imposes fines on vets who support this practice.

- In 2005, the United States Food and Drug Administration announced a ban on the use of the antibiotic enrofloxacin in poultry because it was in the same antibiotic class as ciprofloxacin, used to treat people who have contracted CA-MRSA. One US pharmaceutical company[22] produces both antibiotics.

Zoonotic legacy

Even though we may never have heard of the word 'zoonotic' before, we now need an awareness of the potential transfer of MRSA between humans and animals. We can't turn back time to undo any of the costly mistakes that have been made by farmers, pharmaceutical companies or governments. We are living with this uncomfortable legacy.

Chapter 4

The Evolution of MRSA

Dr Jonathan L Caplin, BSc, PhD, Senior Lecturer
in Microbiology, University of Brighton, UK

MRSA is an acronym for methicillin-resistant *Staphylococcus aureus*, and refers to strains of this bacterium that are resistant to the antibiotic methicillin, and to other members of the beta-lactam class of antibiotics. MRSA is often referred to in the press as a 'superbug', meaning a bacterium resistant to several antibiotics. MRSA infections are classified as either healthcare associated MRSA (HA-MRSA) or community-associated MRSA (CAMRSA), although this distinction is more complicated than simply where the infection was caught. MRSA was first reported in the United Kingdom in 1961[1], and in the United States in 1968.[2] A combination of its virulence, ease of transmission and antibiotic resistance has resulted in MRSA becoming a major problem in the health care setting and in the community.

What are *Staphylococcus aureus* and MRSA?

The name *Staphylococcus*, from the Greek *staphyle*, meaning a bunch of grapes, and *kokkos*, meaning a berry, indicates the appearance of the bacterial cells when viewed using a microscope. It was first described and named in 1880, as the most common cause of abscesses and infected surgical wounds; Louise Pasteur, the French microbiologist, who was the first to grow *S. aureus* in a laboratory, called the resulting bone infections, now known as osteomylitis, a "boil in bone marrow". The bacterium's specific name, *aureus* meaning golden, refers to the golden-yellow colonies (visible clumps of bacteria) it forms on certain laboratory growth media. The full name of this bacterium is often shortened to *Staph. aureus, S. aureus* or sometimes just '*staph*'.

Prior to the development of penicillin in the 1940s, *S. aureus* infections could result in serious and often fatal disease. Most strains of *S. aureus* were sensitive to penicillin, and remarkable recoveries were achieved, but it was soon noted that resistant strains were emerging. By the late 1950s, about 9 out of every 10 *S. aureus* strains isolated from infected patients were penicillin-resistant. A modified form of penicillin called methicillin (also called methicillin), was introduced to treat penicillin-resistant strains, but it needed to be injected and could cause kidney damage, so antibiotics such as oxacillin or flucloxacillin were developed. Resistance to methicillin was first recorded in the 1960s, but did not become a major problem in hospitals until the 1990s.

How did antibiotic resistance develop in *S. aureus*?

Penicillin, and other antibiotics in the same class, kill *S. aureus* by stopping the synthesis of a compound which is an integral part of the bacterial cell wall. This cell wall compound, called peptidoglycan, maintains cell wall integrity, especially in the 'Gram-positive' bacteria. The beta-lactam core of the antibiotic binds to specific sites on the bacterial cell wall, named penicillin-binding proteins, causing disruption of cell wall synthesis. This causes the cell walls to leak or collapse resulting in death of the bacterium.

Antibiotic resistance develops because there are countless different strains of bacteria. If one has a genetic mutation which gives it a survival advantage, such as being resistant to an antibiotic, it will survive, and eventually most strains will carry the resistance genes. There are two mechanisms by which the bacteria develop resistance to penicillin, methicillin and other betalactam antibiotics. Some strains produce an enzyme known as penicillinase, which breaks open the ring structure of the antibiotic, rendering it ineffective. Other strains alter their own proteins so that antibiotics are unable to bind to them and bacterial cell walls are not disrupted.

The evolution of MRSA resulted in strains resistant to penicillin and all beta-lactam antibiotics. MRSA also became resistant to members of the beta-lactam sub group of antibiotics known as the cephalosporins. Recently, strains of MRSA are showing resistance or reduced susceptibility to vancomycin, a member of the glycopeptide class of antibiotics.[3] Since glycopeptide antibiotics are now the drug of choice for severe MRSA infections, the possibility of vancomycin resistance has raised serious concerns regarding successful treatment of multi-drug resistant *Staphlococcus aureus.*

MRSA as a superbug

The world we live in is full of bacteria, the vast majority of which are harmless, although some are more dangerous than others. *S. aureus* is just one of more than 40 species of a large genus of bacteria, and is one of the few *staphylococci* that can cause disease. Like some other species of *staphylococci*, it is a common commensal of humans *i.e.* it comprises part of the body's normal bacterial flora, but without causing disease. *Staphylococci* frequently live on the skin, especially in folds such as the armpit and groin, in the nose and less commonly in the throat.[4] The main mode of transmission from one person to another is via the hands, especially those of healthcare workers. Hands can become contaminated by contact with infected or colonised patients and their wounds, via medical devices, and objects and surfaces contaminated with blood or body fluids containing *S. aureus* or MRSA. Some strains of *S. aureus* can be very resilient and survive for hours, days, or longer on dry surfaces and fabrics. The superbug status of MRSA is further enhanced as several strains have become resistant to many of the disinfectants and antiseptics used in hospitals to clean surfaces, sterilise instruments and decontaminate skin.

MRSA strains give rise to the same diseases and conditions as those caused by antibiotic-sensitive strains, and are usually no more aggressive or infectious. They are only more serious than other *S. aureus* infections because they do not respond to antibiotic treatment. MRSA infections can become more severe than they may otherwise have been if the cause of the infection is not diagnosed early enough, or if prescribed antibiotics do not work. Certain strains of MRSA, particularly those classified as epidemic strains EMRSA-15 and EMRSA-16 (also referred to as ST22 and ST36 respectively), are easily transmissible between patients and hospital staff, and have the capacity to cause serious disease. These strains represent nearly half of the *S. aureus* bloodstream infections (bacteraemia) in England, and about 95% of all bloodstream infections attributed to MRSA.

S. aureus, including MRSA, may cause symptomless colonisation in humans, but is the same bacteria responsible for more serious and potentially life threatening conditions, including bloodstream infections (bacteraemia), endocarditis, pneumonia, scalded skin syndrome, toxic shock syndrome, and necrotizing fasciitis. *S. aureus* can also cause septic arthritis, intravenous line infections, heart-valve infections, urinary tract infections, and some strains are responsible for a type of food poisoning. In severe infections, symptoms can include high fever, raised white blood cell count, rigors (shaking), disturbance of blood clotting with a tendency to bleed into tissue, and the failure of vital organs, often resulting in death. Most of the serious consequences of *S. aureus* infections are a result of one or more virulence factors produced by the bacteria. These include the exotoxins secreted by the bacteria, which act on cell membranes. Other toxins produced by *S. aureus* include exfoliative toxins which cause peeling of the skin, observed with scalded skin syndrome, and enterotoxins, which cause a form of food poisoning. In some strains the golden pigment, staphyloxanthin, acts as a virulence factor, destroying the white blood cells targeting the bacteria.

Treatment of MRSA infections is difficult. Many strains remain sensitive to the antibiotic fusidic acid, but because resistance to it develops easily, it must be used in combination with another antimicrobial for the treatment of serious MRSA infections. For skin infections, topical ointments containing the antibiotic mupirocin are often used, but resistance to this can develop. Mupirocin is bacteriostatic at low doses and bactericidal at high concentrations, and works by inhibiting the synthesis of proteins and RNA (ribonucleic acid), and to a lesser extent, DNA as well as cell wall formation. To treat mupirocin-resistant strains, oral antibiotics such as clindamycin, or a combination of trimethoprim and co-trimoxazole, are being used.[5] Resistance to these antibiotics has led to the use of new, broad spectrum anti-Gram-positive antibiotics such as the oral drug linezolid,[6] and daptomycin.[7] Intravenous vancomycin has become the last resort to treat serious MRSA infections, but it is toxic, and drug levels in blood need regular monitoring. The drug was developed originally for the treatment of infections caused by Gram-positive bacteria such as *S. aureus*, but its side effects outweighed the benefits. Vancomycin still has use in a clinical setting, as many strains remain susceptible to it, but vancomycin-intermediate *S. aureus* (VISA) and vancomycin-resistant *S. aureus* (VRSA) strains have been reported.[8,9]

What is community-associated MRSA (CA-MRSA)?
Although MRSA infections were predominantly found in the hospital or clinical setting (HA-MRSA), there are now an increasing number of outbreaks of MRSA in community settings, in people who were otherwise

healthy, and this has led to the term community-associated MRSA (CA-MRSA) being used. These outbreaks appear to be linked to strains that have some unique properties not seen with HA-MRSA strains. They are usually more virulent and spread more easily, cause skin and soft tissue infections, but are commonly less resistant to antibiotics and easier to treat than HA-MRSA. Some strains of MRSA produce the Panton–Valentine leukocidin (PVL) toxin, which can cause very serious infections.[10] PVL is frequently detected in isolates of CA-MRSA obtained from infections in previously healthy children and young adults.[11] The toxin destroys white blood cells and tissues, causing extensive tissue necrosis and spreading infection. Recent research has demonstrated that over-production of substances termed phenol-soluble modulins (PSMs) could be the main virulence factor in certain strains of CA-MRSA.[12] PSMs are bacterial proteins that can cause a potentially fatal immune reaction called a cytokine storm, which rapidly kills white blood cells and immune cells.

The main criteria differentiating HA-MRSA infections from CA-MRSA infections are that the latter are acquired by persons who have not been hospitalised within the past year, nor undergone invasive medical procedures such as dialysis, surgery, venous or urinary catheterisation. CA-MRSA is most often seen as skin or soft tissue infections (SSTIs) such as boils or abscesses, but can cause more serious health problems, such as blood stream infections or pneumonia. Patients often describe having had what looked like a 'spider bite' before becoming ill. The involved site is red, swollen and painful and may produce yellow pus. The wound may break open or fail to heal and may develop into an abscess. In some cases, CA-MRSA can rapidly lead to widespread and potentially fatal infection.

A number of CA-MRSA strains have been found in the United States, the three most common are named USA-100, USA-300 & USA-400. CA-MRSA strain USA-300 has also been found in England and Wales since at least 2002, where it is called ST8-SCCmec Iva. There is some evidence to suggest that the USA-300 strain is more virulent than other CA-MRSA as it produces the PVL toxin[13] and is commonly found in HIV-infected patients. The USA-300 strain is genetically related to an HA-MRSA strain, which emerged in the 1960s in Europe, after the introduction of methicillin. Both of these strains are thought to be descendants of a methicillin-susceptible ancestral strain.[14]

MRSA and biofilms

Bacteria and other microorganisms can attach to the surface or interface of inanimate objects and develop highly complex structures called biofilms, composed of sticky polymers produced by the bacteria. It has been estimated that biofilms are responsible for more than 80% of all infections, many of which are of nosocomial origin, meaning that they were acquired in a hospital or clinical setting.[15] A common example of a biofilm is the tartar plaque found on teeth. The bacteria within the biofilm matrix interact and function as a unit rather than as individual cells, and chemical signalling processes attract other bacteria. Biofilms offer a protective shield for the microbes, and bacteria in this state are more able to resist antibiotic therapy. Biofilms are a significant problem with catheters, prosthetics, pacemakers, artificial heart valves, dentures and contact lenses.

Many chronic infections caused by *S. aureus* and MRSA are aided by their ability to adhere to medical devices and form a biofilm. When *S. aureus* grows in a biofilm it undergoes an adaptive response. Genetic analysis has identified 48 genes that are induced (switched on) and 84 genes that were repressed (switched off,) during biofilm growth compared to planktonic (free floating) growth.[16] Experiments on the polysaccharide polymers produced by MRSA indicate that biofilm development involves a protein, regulated by genes involved in the adaptive response. Concentrations of carbon dioxide, oxygen and glucose, appear to be triggers for biofilm development, although different mechanisms of biofilm production have been recorded in MSSA and MRSA clinical isolates.[17]

Can MRSA be controlled?

The emergence and increasing occurrence of MRSA, and other antibiotic resistant bacteria, has encouraged the exploration of novel methods of treatment.[18] Laboratory trials with emulsions of nanoparticles coated with a novel, non-water soluble antibiotic, have shown potent activity against MRSA.[19] Pharmaceutical companies are exploring the use of modified versions of older antibiotics and 'cocktails' of antibiotics in the quest to stay one step ahead of the evolving superbug. Laboratory trials of some new antibiotics show promise and there are also attempts to develop immuno-therapies and vaccines specifically against MRSA. The implementation of screening tests to detect MRSA in patients prior to admission for elective surgery, has led to a reduction in hospital infection rates.[20]

MRSA in animals

Not only is MRSA causing a huge problem to human health but it has also spread to animals. It is rare for a disease to cross the species barrier but MRSA can be spread from humans to animals and from animals to humans, and the collective term, zoonosis, has been adopted. The first report of MRSA being isolated from animals was in 1972,[21] and since then, studies suggest that humans were the source of this zoonotic disease, as the isolates are generally the healthcare-associated epidemic strains, EMRSA-15 and EMRSA-16.[22] MRSA has mostly been isolated from dogs and horses, and in some cases, the people associated with the animals. Although the significance of this zoonotic disease in relation to public health has not been fully assessed, there is concern over the increase in the PVL toxin seen in animal-derived *S. aureus* isolates.[23]

Tracking the changes

MRSA is developing at a very fast rate, with mankind desperately trying to catch up, and there is clearly a need for systematic study and vigilance in order to gain control over infection. One initiative, in place since the late 1990s, is a sophisticated surveillance system, under which specialist laboratories in the UK, the USA and Europe collect data on suspected outbreaks of MRSA. This information helps to distinguish between HA-MRSA and CA-MRSA strains, between colonising and infecting isolates, and between new episodes and relapses of infection.[24] Each country forwards its data to a central unit in order for the collective data to be accessible by government departments tracking the spread and evolution of MRSA.

Chapter 5
Microbiology Explained

Professor Valerie Edwards-Jones,
Manchester Metropolitan University, UK

The human body is constantly exposed to thousands of microorganisms. For example, we breathe in approximately 10,000 microorganisms daily but we only succumb to infection if the microorganism can cause disease or when our immune system fails to protect us.

There are four major groups of microorganisms: bacteria, viruses, fungi and parasites. The different groups of microorganism cause different types of disease. Examples of common diseases are shown in table 1.

Microorganism	Example of clinical disease
Bacteria	Diphtheria, tuberculosis, gas gangrene, tetanus, gonorrhea
Virus	Influenza, chicken pox, polio, hepatitis, HIV
Fungi	Thrush, fungal nail infection, ringworm
Parasite	Scabies, head lice, malaria, tapeworm

Examples of different microorganisms and clinical disease

Bacteria, fungi and parasites can live independently outside a human cell whereas viruses live and multiply within a human cell. The different treatments available include:

antibiotics	(for bacterial infections)	e.g. **penicillin**
antifungal agents	(for fungal infections)	e.g. **nyastatin**
antiviral agents	(for viral infections)	e.g. **acyclovir**
antiparasitic agents	(for parasite infections)	e.g. **quinine**

These antimicrobial agents act on specific target sites within the microorganism and because many of those sites are unique to the microorganism and not to a human cell, they can be relatively non-toxic. This is why these antimicrobial agents can be used within the body without causing too many side effects. Some people may be allergic or intolerant to antimicrobial compounds, including antibiotics.

There are other groups of antimicrobial agents that have a more general use to prevent or treat infection, inhibit growth or reduce the numbers of microorganisms. These are disinfectants, antiseptics and preservatives.

Disinfectants can be toxic to human cells so are only used in the environment to reduce numbers of microorganisms on surfaces. The most commonly used, cost-effective home disinfectant is chlorine bleach.

Preservatives are natural or synthetic substances that are added to products such as pharmaceuticals, paints, foods, wood, etc. to prevent decomposition by microorganisms. Natural substances such as salt, sugar, and vinegar are used as traditional preservatives in food products, whereas highly toxic compounds of arsenic, copper and petroleum-based chemical compounds are used in wood preservation.

Antiseptics are substances that can be applied to living tissue or skin to prevent and treat less severe or non-life threatening infections. Many are used for the prevention or treatment of malodour and skin infections. Antiseptics can kill all major groups of microorganisms when used at appropriate concentrations, depending upon the properties of the microorganism, the presence of organic matter, the temperature and the time involved.

Essential oils are nature's antiseptics. Their ability to kill microorganisms has been well documented over the centuries. Hippocrates, the founder of medicine, used aromatic plants as early as 500BC. Essential oils are most commonly extracted from plants of a single botanical source by steam distillation and are known to be a complex mixture of organic hydrocarbons. Essential oil hydrocarbons are volatile organic constituents of the plant matter and have related chemical structures consisting of carbon, hydrogen and oxygen. Chemical analysis of essential oils allows them to be classified depending upon the nature and ratio of components in the oil and this significant difference in chemical composition is what gives each of them their unique properties.

Hydrocarbons consist of isoprene units that make up the terpenes that give the essential oils some of their antiseptic properties.

Terpenes are classified as:

Monoterpenes, which have 2 isoprene units (10 carbon atoms) and

Sesquiterpenes, which have 3 isoprene units (15 carbon atoms). Sesquiterpenes are less common but are major components in some oils, for example in chamomile oil.

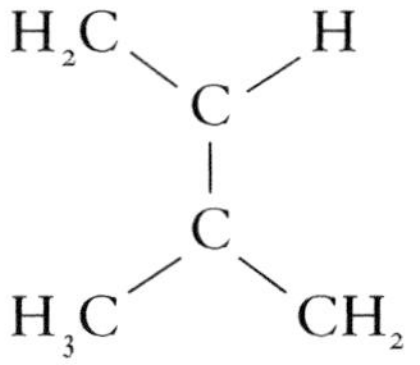

$$H_2C \diagdown C \diagup H$$
$$|$$
$$C$$
$$H_3C \diagup \diagdown CH_2$$

Fig. 1 Chemical structure of an isoprene unit.

Each essential oil has major and minor components. Sometimes the same species of plant can give rise to slightly different ratios of the major components depending upon the environment the plants were grown in and the nature of the soil. These are known as **chemotypes**. There are chemotypes of thyme oil with some rich in thymol, and other chemotypes rich in linalool. Every chemotype could have differing antiseptic properties based on differences in the chemistry.

The most well documented essential oil used as an antiseptic is tea tree oil *(Melaleuca alternifolia)*. It is used in products ranging from hair shampoo and body wash to medicinal formulations such as an after-burn gel for reducing pain and infection.

Determining antimicrobial activity in the laboratory

The antimicrobial activity of an essential oil is determined in the laboratory *(in vitro)* by a number of standard methods. One of the commonest methods employed in the laboratory is the **zone of inhibition (ZOI)** test. This is a very quick and easy method where a standard number of microorganisms (about 1 million bacterial cells per millilitre) are applied to the surface of an agar plate which allows bacteria to grow. A measured amount of essential oil is added either to a

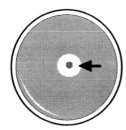

Fig. 2 Zone of Inhibition of bacterial growth indicates activity of antimicrobial product (see Plate 1).

paper disk or to a 'well' bored into the agar. The components in the oil will diffuse into the culture medium and a circular zone will be visible if there is any antimicrobial activity. This is shown in figure 2, indicated by the arrow. Unfortunately the size of the zone of inhibition is not proportional to its activity as essential oils contain up to one hundred different chemicals, each with its own diffusion properties. Therefore any zone is used as an indicator of antimicrobial activity.

Another common method used for testing essential oils is using the **minimum inhibitory concentration (MIC)** test. The MIC is determined by diluting the essential oil to levels that may be used safely on the human skin. Essential oils for skin massage are normally used at a maximum concentration of 2% unless prescribed in a more concentrated form for a specific reason. A 2% dilution is generally the highest concentration tested. A series of dilutions is made in culture medium - a nutritious broth that will allow bacteria under test to grow - that ranges from the maximum to the lowest concentration, for example 2%, 1%, 0.5%, 0.25%, 0.125%, 0.06%, and 0.03%. Once the dilution series is made, bacteria are added to each concentration and incubated at 37°C overnight. The MIC is determined as the lowest concentration inhibiting growth. This is shown below in figure 3.

Microbial growth is usually determined by the turbidity created by the growing cells. The tubes where growth occurs are those that have had very low concentrations of the essential oils added. When a higher concentration has been used no growth is observed. However, sometimes when essential oils are diluted into the aqueous culture

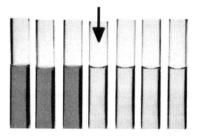

Fig. 3 The first tube where there is no growth, indicated by the arrow, is the MIC (see Plate 2).

medium, the essential oil does not disperse fully and creates an 'emulsion' or 'sol', creating a false turbidity. Occasionally the essential oil 'floats' on the surface of the aqueous medium. A surfactant (e.g. Tween 20: 0.5%) can be added to the aqueous medium to help with the dispersion of the essential oil, helping to negate this.

The **minimum bactericidal concentration (MBC)** is then determined by sub-culturing the tubes where no growth is observed. A loopful (a standard laboratory measurement) of the broth is sub-cultured onto fresh culture media by streaking across the surface of a nutrient agar plate. The concentration where no growth is observed following sub-culture is called the MBC. When using essential oils the MIC and the MBC are often the same. Once the MBC has been determined, the time taken to kill the microorganism can then be ascertained. The MBC is created in a broth and known numbers of the microorganism added, at time denoted ohr. At set time intervals, usually 15 minutes, 30 minutes, 1hr, 2hr, 4hr, 8hr and 24hr, a sample is taken and the numbers of microorganisms accurately counted. The time taken to reduce the numbers to nil is known as the killing time or the time-kill. It is also important to be aware of the numbers of microorganisms added to the test system, as the initial concentration of the numbers of microorganisms can affect the efficiency of killing. The standard methods for these tests can be found in the British Standard testing methods or the European Standard testing methods.[1]

Reported antimicrobial activity of essential oils

In a study carried out by Hammer and Carson in 2000, the MIC/MBC of tea tree oil (*Melaleuca alternifolia*) was compared to prescribed antifungal agents ketoconazole, miconazole and econazole, which are used to treat the fungus *Malassezia* spp. that causes a skin condition known as *Psityrias versiculor*. Tea tree oil, at a range of 0.12% - 0.25% was comparable to ketoconazole. Other studies have shown that tea tree oil can inhibit a wide range of bacteria, some of which are resistant to commonly used antibiotics. The analysis of tea tree oil has shown that the major terpenes/ sesquiterpines are terpinen-4-ol (38%), gamma-terpinene (20%), alphaterpinene (10%), 1, 8-cineole (4%) and alpha-pinene (5%). These are also the major antimicrobial components.

These individual components that make up the whole essential oil can be antimicrobial in their own right. Sometimes, they are more active than the parent essential oil but, individually, are often more toxic than when combined in the parent oil. The two major components from tea tree oil, 1, 8 cineol (eucalyptol) and terpinen-4-ol, both have very good antimicrobial properties.

How do essential oils work as antimicrobial agents?

Tea tree oil, as an example, disrupts the cell membrane of the bacterium, causing a loss of potassium ions from the cell. The lipophilic (lipid loving) monoterpenes integrate with the phospholipids in the membrane and leakage occurs. Antimicrobial essential oils have also been known to cause inhibition of glucose dependant respiration in *S. aureus*, *E. coli* and *C. albicans*.

Some common essential oils with antiseptic properties are:

- Tea tree oil *(Melaleuca alternifolia)*

- Geranium oil *(Pelargonium graveolens)*

- Lavender oil *(Lavandula angustifolia)*

Antimicrobial activity in vaporised form

One of the most noticeable things about essential oils is their aroma. Some of the fragrant parts of the essential oil are also antimicrobial. The vapours released from essential oils have been proven to be highly antimicrobial. A recent study has shown that MRSA and *Clostridium difficle* have been killed in the laboratory by a blend of vapours released from a variety of dispersion devices. The most efficient system is the use of 'venturi technology' where air is forced over the surface

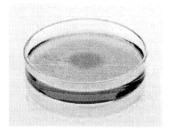

Fig. 4   Zone of Inhibition plate. The cleared central area is where the essential oil has destroyed the bacteria (see Plate 3).

of essential oil blends and antimicrobial vapours are released into the atmosphere, killing bacteria in the air as well as on the surface. This use of essential oils is extremely exciting for reducing the spread of airborne healthcare associated infections.

In summary, essential oils have a huge potential for exploitation in the healthcare setting. Many of the bacteria we now see routinely in hospitals are resistant to many antibiotics. Alternative treatments have to be found. Essential oils offer a new direction in the prevention and treatment of infectious disease in the future.

Part Two
ANTIMICROBIAL ESSENTIAL OILS

This part of the book looks specifically at those essential oils scientifically proven to possess antibacterial activity, and aims to relay this information in a simple way. A vast amount of microbiology research over the last few decades has been able to show which oils will inhibit growth of bacteria (bacteriostatic) and which are able to kill bacteria (bactericidal).

Chapter 6

Tea Tree

Tea tree oil was, just two decades ago, virtually unknown outside of Australia. Today it is a household name, in almost every country in the developed world. The popularity of tea tree is due to its wide-ranging healing properties. It is known as 'a medicine chest in a bottle'. Many books have been written about the versatility of tea tree oil and many more health books contain a mention, or even a profile on tea tree. This chapter will look specifically at the antimicrobial propeties of tea tree oil and the scientific papers written and published in respected journals. A great deal of microbiology research has been conducted with tea tree oil but the microbe of interest to this book is the bacterium *Staph aureus*.

Tea tree (*Melaleuca alternifolia*)

Geographical location: South Eastern Australia, notably the swampy, subtropical coastal region of New South Wales, although it is being cultivated in other parts of the continent. Tea tree, since its rise in popularity, has been successfully grown in Zimbabwe, Kenya, China, Vietnam, India and Guatemala. Chinese tea tree is now competing with Australian tea tree in the international essential oils marketplace.

The difference between tea tree and manuka

Tea tree comes from the same botanical family as New Zealand manuka, which is also known as the New Zealand ti tree, but there the similarity ends. Although both plants are from the *Myrtacaea* family, the shape, size, aroma and chemistry are widely different. Tea tree is known to be toxic if taken internally in anything other than the tiny amount found in toothpaste or mouth wash. This in itself differentiates it from manuka, the plant that gives rise to manuka honey. A commercially available Jellybush honey is being marketed as Tea Tree Honey, but Jellybush is not a melaleuca. It is *Leptospermum polygalifolium*, one of the seventy nine species of *Leptospermum* in Australia. All are overshadowed by their famous New Zealand relative, manuka.

Habitat

Over three hundred varieties of *Melaleuca* grow throughout Australia and the most well known is *Melaleuca alternifolia*, which thrives naturally in the north eastern region of New South Wales. There, the tea trees growing in the swampy area of Bungawalbyn Creek have been harvested for over sixty years. This product is known as Bush Oil. Today the majority of tea tree oil is grown in plantations. Tea trees require a lot of moisture and plantations have to be very well irrigated.

M. alternifolia is a small, five to seven metre tall, tree or shrub, with needlelike leaves similar to cyprus or rosemary. It grows prolifically across south eastern Australia. The aroma-chemistry changes from the south to the north of its natural habitat. Trees in the south produce high levels of 1,8-cineole and good levels of terpinen-4-ol. Trees in the north produce high terpinen-4-ol with lower levels of 1,8-cineole.

Tea trees produce tiny white flowers in the spring. Essential oil is produced in the summer season, which in Australia is between December and May. There is rapid growth during the summer months and less in the winter months. The essential oil is a pale yellow-green or clear liquid with a distinctive aroma: warm, spicy and camphoraceous.

Melaleuca linariifolia, also called 'Snow in Summer', is a native of eastern Australia. As with *M. alternifolia*, it grows near watercourses or swamps, but can reach heights of up to 10 metres. Its bark is like paper, which is why it is known as one of the Australian 'paper bark' trees.

Melaleuca dissitiflora, commonly known as Creek tea tree, is another paper bark. It grows to a height of 5 metres and is a native of Western Australia, South Australia, Northern Territory and Queensland.

The plant and its products

The tea tree is valued for its essential oil. In order to keep up with industry demand, a great many tea tree plantations have been set up in several areas of the country. At the end of the twentieth century, Australia was producing between 300 to 400 tonnes a year, and planning to increase output to 1,000 tonnes, but in the early part of the twenty-first century Chinese tea tree became commercially available. This has had a negative effect on Australian tea tree production as many growers were unable to compete with the lower Chinese prices and switched to growing other crops.

The benefits of tea tree have been known to the indigenous aboriginals for many hundreds of years, but the myriad of uses for its essential oil, and the potential of tea tree oil as a commercial product, has been recognised for barely a century. Tea tree is known to be antiseptic, antibacterial, antifungal, anti-viral and anti-inflammatory. Tea tree essential oil is analysed and graded before being offered for sale.

Superior grade is the highest priced tea tree oil and is incorporated into medicinal products for human and animal use. It must offer a minimum terpinen-4-ol content of 35% and contain a maximum of 5% cineole. One pharmaceutical preparation with tea tree is an emergency dressing for burns. It comes in sterile packs ready for use by ambulance crews.

Standard grade has a slightly different ratio of aroma-chemistry, containing between 30% to 35% terpinen-4-ol and up to 8% cineole.

Industrial grade tea tree oil contains lower levels of terpinen-4-ol and variable levels of cineole and is used for disinfectants and detergents.

Chemistry of tea tree

The chemical make up of tea tree essential oil varies considerably depending on its habitat. As far back as the 1930's, researchers[1] had analysed the aroma-chemicals and made a declaration that trees producing high levels of cineole, in the 20% to 40% range, were of less importance than trees with high terpinen-4-ol and low cineole levels. Cineole was considered to be inactive, even though it is a normal component of tea tree, and had been employed for its germicidal activity since 1925.

Tea tree oil is a complex mixture of terpenes and terpene-alcohols. A typical batch analysis would show over a hundred components, with 90% of the oil content made up of the following: terpinen-4-ol, 1,8-cineole, alpha-terpineol, terpinolene, alpha & gamma terpinene. The main antimicrobial component, and therefore the most valued component, is the terpinen-4-ol.

Over the years, most Australian commercial plantations have made the decision to cultivate tea trees with 1,8-cineole levels ranging from 4% to 10% and with terpinen-4-ol levels within a 30% to 40% ratio. This is in keeping with the current Australian Government Standard which specifies that tea tree oil should contain not more than 15% 1,8-cineole, and that the major active ingredient, terpinen-4-ol, must be at least 30%. When these ratios were set it was believed that cineole inhibited the antimicrobial action of terpinen-4-ol.

Australian Standard 1997 — AS 2782 (ISO 4730:1996)

In 1985, the Australian Standard stated that the name of *Melaleuca alternifolia* could be given to a tea tree oil provided that it met their parameter of at least 30% of terpinen-4-ol and a maximum of 15% cineole and that any of the three hundred tea tree varieties could be included in the mix. The new Standard of 1997, replacing the 1985 standard, specifies that only three tea trees should be used: *Melaleuca alternifolia, Melaleuca linariifolia* and *Melaleuca dissitiflora,* and that the resultant blend can still be called tea tree with the INCI name of *Melaleuca alternifolia,* as long as the minimum/ maximum levels of the key components are met. This means that even when a tea tree oil is labeled as 'organic' it could still be a blend of the three *Melaleucas,* as long as each of them are grown organically. There are also tea tree plantations producing tea tree oil exclusively from cloned *Melaleuca alternifolia.*

According to the 1997 Australian Standard: Oil of *Melaleuca,* terpinen-4-ol type, tea tree oil "may be obtained by steam distillation of the foliage and terminal branchlets of:

- *Melaleuca alternifolia,*
- *Melaleuca linariifolia,*
- *Melaleuca dissitiflora,*
- As well as other species of *Melaleuca*

provided that the oil obtained conforms to the requirements given in this International Standard."

In 1993, research[2] to determine the optimum ratio of aroma chemicals in tea tree produced some interesting end results. The experiment was to show whether or not cineole, in excess of the specified maximum levels of 15%, would inhibit the antimicrobial action of terpinen-4-ol. The research team carried out a series of tests with *Staphylococcus aureus*, and other microbes, using tea tree oil with added cineole, and with blending cineole with terpinen-4-ol in varying ratios. The addition of cineole in concentrations of up to 30% was seen to be synergistic rather than antagonistic, as long as the terpinen-4-ol levels did not fall below 30%.

There was a decrease in antimicrobial effectiveness but only when terpinen-4-ol levels fell below 30%. The conclusion was: "that greater antimicrobial activity for tea tree oil is not achieved by increasing terpinen-4-ol concentrations above 40%, nor by decreasing cineole levels below 40%, provided that terpinen-4-ol remains at approximately 30% to 45%. Consequently optimal bioactivity can be achieved with cineole present at 20% to 40% as long as terpinen-4-ol is maintained at 25% to 40%."

With all of its documented germicidal and healing properties, tea tree has, over the past few years, been accused of being a skin irritant. Research[3] has been conducted with skin patch testing. Results showed that less than 1% of volunteers reported any negative effects. Possible theories for the slight irritancy are that fresh tea tree does not cause any problems but that oxidized tea tree is potentially problematic. According to one commercial manufacturer of tea tree products[4] it is the para-cymene content of tea tree that creates skin irritancy in a small number of users. This chemical can be present in tea tree between 2% and 12%. Para-cymene is documented as being non-toxic, but is known to be a mild to moderate skin irritant. The company uses a tea tree strain that is low in para-cymene for its skincare products. These facts have been backed up by research[5] published in Contact Dermatology.

Microbiology research with tea tree oil

Tea tree is one of the most-researched essential oils. Studies over several years have looked at its efficacy against a number of microorganisms.

Research into the antimicrobial status of tea tree goes back to 1923 when Dr Penfold[6] looked at the way tea tree oil killed bacteria and declared that tea tree oil was thirteen times stronger as a bactericide than carbolic acid. He presented his findings in 1925, to the Royal Society of New South Wales.

More recent investigation[7] looked into the level of antimicrobial activity of each of the major components of tea tree oil and concluded that it was the alcohols such as terpinen-4-ol that were the most antimicrobial. The research also compared terpinen-4-ol extracted from tea tree oil with tea tree oil, and found that against *Staph aureus* they were equally efficient.

The researchers realized that when it comes to killing off *Staph aureus* in laboratory tests, it is the wide range of components in tea tree oil that contributes to the antimicrobial activity, and that a higher level of terpinen-4-ol may not necessarily increase the oil's antimicrobial activity.

One microbiology study[8] looked at the antimicrobial activity of several Australasian essential oils: tea tree, Australian lavender, New Zealand manuka, lemongrass and eucalyptus. Tea tree was found to occupy the middle position in order of antimicrobial activity.

When individual aroma chemicals were compared to tea tree in zone of inhibition tests with *Staph aureus* the results were as follows:

Linalool	16.0 mm
Tea tree	15.0 mm
Terpinen-4-ol	14.0 mm
Lavender	12.5 mm
Linalyl acetate	4.5 mm

These figures represent the millimeters of *Staph aureus* killed in a Petri dish.

The study challenged several different microorganisms with the above aromatic liquids. It found that manuka was inferior to tea tree for the majority, but that for the organism *Staph aureus* there was no difference between the antimicrobial activity of standard tea tree oil and the manuka oil from East Cape region of New Zealand.

This 1998 research study also conducted microbiology trials with various ratios of tea tree and manuka oil against *Staph aureus*, looking at the relative antimicrobial activity in zone of inhibition tests:

Standard tea tree (30% terpinen-4-ol)	10.5 mm
Manuka	9.5 mm
Tea tree oil + Manuka in a ratio of 3:1	10.0 mm
Tea tree oil + Manuka in a ratio of 1:3	10.0 mm

In 1995, further research[9] took place in Australia to analyse the antimicrobial effects of the major components of tea tree oil. The results were as follows:

1,8-cineole	no recorded activity
terpinen-4-ol	active against all test organisms including *Staph aureus*
para-cymene	no antimicrobial activity
linalool	active against several organisms including *Staph aureus*
alpha-terpineol	active against several organisms including *Staph aureus* & that alpha-terpineol was an important synergistic influence on the antimicrobial kill effects of tea tree oil.

Interestingly, the researchers concluded that although terpinen-4-ol is identified as being the main antimicrobial substance in tea tree oil, when used on its own it was less effective at killing *Staph aureus*, and that alpha-terpineol had an important synergistic influence on the antimicrobial effects of tea tree oil.

In zone of inhibition tests, they found terpinen-4-ol to have a kill zone of 6.9 mm and that the kill zone for tea tree was 7.9 mm.

An independent researcher[10], working with tea tree as an antimicrobial agent, found that increasing the level of terpinen-4-ol above a certain level did not enhance the antimicrobial effects.

Researchers in a London hospital[11] carried out time-kill studies with the standard tea tree oil (30% terpinen-4-ol) and tea tree oil with increased concentrations of terpinen-4-ol (superior tea tree oil) in order to determine whether one was any more effective than the other.

Both tea tree oils were tested against a wide range of microorganisms, isolated from bacteria taken from hospital patients. Amongst the microorganisms were methicillin sensitive *Staph aureus* (MSSA) and methicillin resistant/vancomycin tolerant (MRSA). A 5% concentration of each tea tree oil was used. It was found that MRSA isolates were killed more slowly than the MSSA isolates and that the standard tea tree oil was less effective than the superior oil.

Clinical trials with tea tree oil

Since the turn of the new century several clinical trials have been undertaken to prove that tea tree oil is an effective agent in decolonising MRSA. Other trials have been set up to disprove the prevailing conception that tea tree oil is a skin irritant.

In Perth, Australia, the Australian Society for Microbiology hosted "2001: A Microbial Odyssey."[12] The conference had speakers on various aspects of microbial control and included talks on viral conditions such as herpes, the fungal condition candida, as well as presentations from tea tree researchers who had been instrumental in the setting up of clinical trials. They had compared the effect of tea tree oil with the standard mupirocin treatment used for clearing MRSA from carriers. One speaker[13] from the University of Western Australia said: "A pilot study of thirty MRSA carriers comparing routine mupirocin nasal ointment and triclosan skin wash with tea tree oil ointment and wash, showed one third were completely cleared by tea tree but only 13% by conventional treatment."

In 2003, a study was set up in a Sydney institute[14] to assess the risk of dermatitis occurring amongst people using tea tree oil. Patch testing was carried out using varying concentrations of tea tree oil in several different bases. Dilutions tested were 5%, 25% and 100% and test sites were assessed every 48 hours to determine whether sensitisation had occurred. At the end of the trial period it was found that out of three hundred people, only three had experienced an allergic reaction. The overall results were zero allergic reactions at a 5% tea tree dilution and 0.25% allergic reactions at 100% tea tree oil.

Further research to compare tea tree oil with the standard topical antibiotic mupirocin was published in 2003.[15] The purpose was to compare two methods of eliminating MRSA from the nose, where it can be carried by hospital patients who could then infect themselves, and from body sites where MRSA bacteria can be harboured. The standard treatment was a 2% mupirocin nasal cream used in conjunction with a triclosan body wash. The tea tree regimen used a 4% tea tree oil ointment for use in the nose plus a body wash with 5% tea tree oil. At the end of the trial period the researchers concluded: "the tea tree oil products appeared to work as well as the standard hospital treatments."

In 2004, a paper[16] was published on a clinical trial carried out in the UK. The randomised control trial compared the efficacy of tea tree preparations to a standard hospital regimen for the eradication of MRSA colonisation.

The standard regimen comprised the topical antibiotic mupirocin in a 2% dilution, for nasal treatment, along with chlorhexidine and a silver infiltrated cream for cleansing colonised body sites. The tea tree regimen consisted of a 10% tea tree cream and 5% tea tree in a body wash. One hundred people were involved in the five-day trial with the standard regimen, and by the end 49% were cleared. A similar number of people were treated with the tea tree products and 47% were cleared. The trial conclusion was that whilst the topical antibiotic was more effective at clearing nasal carriage of MRSA, the tea tree products worked better at clearing the colonised body sites.

In 2005, a paper was published[17] into the efficacy of using tea tree oil in hand cleansing formulations. The activity of different concentrations of tea tree oil, a hygienic hand wash, an alcoholic hygienic skin wash and an alcohol-based hand rub were investigated. *Staph aureus* and three other bacteria were significantly reduced within one-minute contact time.

A three-year trial, which started in 2007, and was completed in 2010, was reported in a UK medical journal[18] under the title "Doctors test tea tree oil body wash for MRSA". The trial was set up to see if tea tree oil in a body wash could be used to prevent critically ill, hospitalized adults from becoming infected with MRSA. A 5% tea tree preparation was used daily for washing patients in intensive care units, whilst baby soap was used for daily washing of patients in the control group. Research results had not been published at time of *Aromatherapy vs MRSA* going to print.

Contra-indications

- Tea tree oil should not be taken internally as some of the naturally occuring aroma-chemicals can exert a depressant effect. (Tea tree contains aroma-chemicals which are also found in eucalyptus leaves, the staple diet of the permanently intoxicated koala).

- In a minority of cases tea tree oil may induce skin irritancy. If this happens, its use should be discontinued and an alternative, replacement essential oil found.

- It is best to avoid using the neat oil during pregnacy and lactation, although products containing small amounts of tea tree oil, for body/ hair care or for localised treatment of cuts and scratches etc., are considered safe.

- Some cat owners have reported adverse effects from use of tea tree products. However, veterinary practitioners knowledgeable in the use of essential oils, regularly use tea tree oil with good results.

Chapter 7
Manuka

Manuka honey has become very popular over the last few years and its popularity has much to do with its reputation as a remarkable health food with antibacterial properties. Manuka bushes contain an essential oil, and although the link is not yet proven, it is probable that the antimicrobial essential oil in the plant is what ultimately gives manuka honey its antibacterial activity. This chapter will look at manuka honey as well as the essential oil, but first it will take a look at the difference between manuka and kanuka. There has been some confusion between the two, with some people thinking that they are one and the same plant.

Manuka (*Leptospermum scoparium*)

Geographical location: South & North Islands, New Zealand. Some manuka plants also grow in Eastern & Western Australia, New Guinea and Southeast Asia.

Kanuka (*Kunzea ericoides*)

Geographical location: South & North Islands, New Zealand. South Australia, Victoria, New South Wales, Queensland.

The difference between Manuka and Kanuka

Kanuka is often confused with manuka, and although they are from the same *Myrtaceae* family, along with Australian tea tree, they are very different plants with distinctively different aroma-chemistry. Manuka is commonly called the New Zealand ti-tree, although it looks nothing like its Australian relative, and its chemical composition is unique. There is a visual similarity between kanuka and manuka as both plants produce flowers with five white petals surrounding a dark red centre. Manuka flowers are spaced singly on the stems, whilst kanuka flowers grow in clusters along the stems. The size of the blossoms also varies, manuka being 8 mm to 12 mm in diameter whilst kanuka are much smaller, at 3 mm to 5 mm in diameter. The chemical compostion of the two plants also sets them apart, with kanuka plants containing none of the triketones found in manuka. The aroma–chemistry of kanuka does have antibacterial properties but it has been found to be significantly less potent than manuka.

Manuka

Manuka grows prolifically right across New Zealand, from coastal areas to the upper regions of the hills. It is a fast growing plant with an average height of four metres, but varies from a ground level shrub to an eight metre tall tree. Manuka plants are subject to seasonal variations in temperature. Throughout New Zealand the flowering times fall between September and February with the peak flowering time between November and January.

After the flowering season is over and the bees have returned to their hives to make honey, the harvesting of leaves and small branches begins. These parts of the shrub contain a valuable essential oil. The cut material is allowed to wilt before being distilled with high pressure steam passing through the distillation vessels. According to the New Zealand Crop & Food Research Centre manuka oil takes between two to six hours to distill, as the aroma–chemicals (sesquiterpenes) in manuka are heavier than the aroma–chemicals found in the majority of aromatic plants, including kanuka, which contains mostly monoterpenes.

The plant & its products

The essential oil of manuka has a yellow to light brown colour with a taste and aroma described as honey–like, with a sharp but earthy flavour. The oil is widely used in the perfume and toiletries industries.

Manuka honey is an important industry to New Zealand. A great deal of research has already been done, and continues to be done, in order to regulate the describing and naming of the varying grades of manuka honey.

Medicinal grade manuka honey is incorporated into wound dressings and topical agents and these are increasingly being used to heal chronic wounds in hospitals around the world.

Chemistry of manuka oil and how it changes with location

The essential oil distilled from manuka plants varies in aroma, chemical constituents and antibacterial potency according to where the plant was grown. Researchers in New Zealand have grouped manuka essential oils into three main chemotypes, and the following information is courtesy of the New Zealand Crop & Food Research Centre.

A high pinene content is to be found in the northern end of the North Island.

A high triketone content is to be found in the East Cape area of the North Island and also in the Marlborough Sounds area of the South Island. Triketones are the three ketones: leptospermone, iso–leptospermone and flavesone.

A complex mix of aroma-chemicals is to be found in manuka plants growing over the rest of New Zealand.

Research has demonstrated that the triketones in manuka are responsible for its high antibacterial action, which is why the geographical area is of so much interest.

Across New Zealand it has been found that the important triketone chemistry falls roughly as follows, although even plants in one area can vary in composition.

	Triketones
East Cape of North Island	20% – 33%
Marlborough Sounds area of South Island	15% – 20%
East Cape (North Island) & Marlborough Sounds	10% – 15%
Marlborough Sounds and most of the North Island	5% – 10%
Most of South Island	5% or less

Current research is being conducted by Dr. M. Leach of the Crop & Food Research Institute of New Zealand to identify climatic and environmental conditions that influence the value of UMF in honeys. A study will also be done into the potential of breeding specific manuka cultivars.

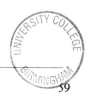

Research with manuka oil

Over the past decade or so, a considerable amount of microbiology research has gone into looking at the potential of manuka essential oil as an effective antibacterial and possible substitute for antibiotics. It is interesting to see conflicting, yet useful, results. This is possibly due to researchers using manuka oils with varying levels of triketones.

In 1994, researchers[1] investigated the action of manuka and kanuka oils. They used fifteen strains of *Staph aureus*, other Gram-positive and Gram-negative bacteria, as well as other organisms. Results showed manuka to have the highest activity against Gram-positive organisms, recorded at approximately twenty times that of tea tree. Kanuka was similar in its action to tea tree. When tested against Gram-negative bacteria, kanuka and manuka were similar in their action, both two to three times less effective than tea tree.

Research in 1998[2], conducted to compare the antibacterial properties of Australian tea tree, Australian lavender, New Zealand manuka, lemongrass and eucalyptus oils, found that the outcome depended on the bacteria under review. Although each essential oil had some antimicrobial properties, the activity varied according to which microorganisms were tested. Manuka oil from the East Cape, high in triketones, was found to have the strongest antimicrobial action against the Gram-positive MRSA.

In 1999, research[3] was undertaken to compare the antimicrobial effects of Australian tea tree with a selection of Australasian essential oils from the *Myrtaceae* family: cajeput, eucalyptus, kanuka, manuka and niaouli. Overall, the highest antimicrobial activity was with tea tree oil, with the exception of the Gram-positive bacteria, for which a higher activity was recorded with manuka.

Research[4] in 2000, looked at the antimicrobial action of essential oils from a range of 'tea trees': Australian tea tree, cajuput, niaouli, kanuka and manuka, along with the b-triketone complex isolated from manuka. Results, once again, showed that manuka oil had the best overall effect against Gram-positive bacteria.

However, in 2001, research[5] concluded that: "Kanuka and manuka oils as well as the b-triketone complex (the active principle of manuka) lacked any bactericidal properties. Their high effectiveness against Gram–positive bacteria can be explained by their bacteriostatic effects." It was observed that the oils tested proved to inhibit bacterial growth, but had not actively killed the bacteria. An extract of manuka oil, composed mainly of triketones, when blended with tea tree oil, had the most powerful bacteriacidal effect, prompting further research.

In the same year, 2001, a larger team of researchers[6] took the active aroma-chemicals, b-triketone complex from manuka oil, and mixed them with tea tree oil. They then made a mix of niaouli (*Melaleuca viridiflora*) with the b-triketone complex. Against four different bacteria, including *Staph aureus*, both blends acheived a complete kill within 240 minutes.

Further research[7] in 2001, looked at the bacterial effect of a blend of Austalian tea tree and New Zealand manuka essential oils. When the blend had more manuka than tea tree, the mixture was more effective against Gram-positive organisms such as *Staph aureus*. Conversely, when the mixture had a higher proportion of tea tree to manuka, the mixture was more effective against Gram–negative organisms such as *E. coli*.

Although the majority of manuka research has been with honey, the triketone research findings show how potent the essential oil can be against *Staphlococcus aureus* and MRSA.

Honey

Honey is a saturated solution of sugars and has been used to heal wounds for hundreds of years. The presence of honey in a deep wound enables the wound to stay open, yet filled with honey, bacteria is prevented from getting in, and healing can take place from the inside out. Healing of a wound can only occur when the infection has been eliminated, and by using honey, bacterial growth can be inhibited whilst the body repairs the damaged flesh. Honey consists of water and sugars, with approximately 15% water to 85% sugars. It is well known that bacteria can readily breed in water, but not easily in honey. Honey is similar to salt, in that it has the ability to draw water to itself by osmosis, and therefore by drawing water from a wound it draws bacteria with it. Honey is acidic with a pH value range of 3.2 to 4.5. This is a contributing factor to honey's antimicrobial action on the skin, which has a pH of 5.

The first indication that the antimicrobial activity of honey was not just an osmotic effect was in a report published in 1919.[8] Researchers observed that the antibacterial potency was increased by limited dilution of honey. Two decades later, research[9] led to the identification of an antibacterial factor which was named 'inhibine'. This term was used in research literature for the next twenty-six years until the antibacterial factor was identified as hydrogen peroxide.[10] This is formed when the bee injects an enzyme (glucose oxidase) into the nectar it has collected during the process of making honey. The glucose oxidase is damaged when honey is heated and the honey loses much of its antibacterial properties. Honey is sensitive to heat and light and must be carefully stored to avoid loss of its glucose oxidase activity.

Recent findings by Professor Molan, leading expert in the field of honey and manuka research, are included in a book[11] published in 2009: "The clearance of infection by honey may involve more than the antibacterial activity of honey, as research findings with leukocytes in cell culture indicate that honey may also work by stimulating the activity of the immune system." And: "The use of hydrogen peroxide as an antiseptic has been discouraged because it is cytotoxic, but at the low levels that form in honey this is not a problem. Many antiseptics in common use, including silver, are cytotoxic and slow the healing process. Honey is not only nontoxic but stimulates the growth of cells involved in wound healing."

As most honeys contain spores of *Clostridium botulinum*, there is some concern about using honey in wounds. For this reason, honey used for commercially manufactured, impregnated dressings for topical use is always sterilized, not by heat but by gamma-irradiation.

Honey is a potent remedy for treating infected wounds because of its levels of acidity, its osmolarity and its hydrogen peroxide activity which increases when it comes into contact with fluid in the wound. Manuka honey has all these antibacterial qualities, but in addition, it has something that has been called Unique Manuka Factor (UMF), differentiating manuka from other honeys.

Manuka honey
Manuka honeys are classified by their strength against bacteria. It was Waikato University in New Zealand that first discovered that manuka

honey had an antibacterial agent in addition to the hydrogen peroxide activity. The discovery was made by an MSc student[12] in 1982, but it was not until 1988, after much further investigation by Professor Molan and a team of researchers that a scientific paper was published[13] on the nonperoxide activity of manuka honey. This research concluded: "It was found that in the honeys with high antibacterial activity, a larger part of this activity was due to a factor other than hydrogen peroxide. The test microorganism used, *Staphylococcus aureus*, was not inhibited by the osmolarity or the acidity of the honey. The association of high antibacterial activity with particular floral sources suggests that the non-peroxide antibacterial activity is of floral origin."

UMF – Unique Manuka Factor

Unique Manuka Factor rating is set by the Active Manuka Honey Association (AMHA). In a microbiology laboratory, batches of manuka honey are challenged with *Staphylococcus aureus* and the results compared with similar tests using phenol, a carbolic acid once used as a disinfectant. It is a powerful germicide and was the active ingredient found in traditional antiseptics such as TCP, commonly used for disinfecting cuts and scrapes. The number that follows the trade mark UMF is equal to the concentration of phenol used, indicating that the same strength of antibacterial activity is present in the honey. So, a manuka honey with a UMF10 rating would be equal to a 10% dilution of phenol, whilst a UMF20 rating would be equal to a 20% dilution of phenol, which would be twice as strong.

The UMF standard was established to identify and set apart from other manuka honey, those manuka honeys which had the mysterious 'non-hydrogen peroxide' antibacterial activity. Such honey can be diluted 10-fold or more and still completely inhibit the usual wound-infecting microorganisms.

Where honey is diluted by body fluid, the acidity of honey makes a minor contribution to antibacterial activity. It is the other antibacterial components that are primarily responsible for control of infection when honey is used therapeutically. Some phenolic acid components of manuka honey have been identified, but these comprise just 4% of its non-hydrogen peroxide antibacterial activity. The unusual antibacterial activity in manuka honey is fully effective, even when it is undiluted.

Manuka honey manufacturers analyse every batch of honey as it comes from bee-keepers in each of the manuka honey producing areas, and then blend the batches together, in specific ratios, in order to produce 'industry standard' manuka UMF10, manuka UMF15, manuka UMF20 and higher. These high potency honeys are often used for the treatment of MRSA infected wounds, even though the honey is not irradiated. The recommendation is to use CE regulated medical honey products to treat MRSA-infected wounds. Honey that is UMF5 is not considered powerful enough to treat MRSA.

Outside of New Zealand, an entirely different method of establishing and measuring the antibacterial activity of manuka honey was discovered by German reseachers in 2006.[14] Since that time there has been much interest in the measurement of methyl-glyoxal. It is naturally produced in humans, animals and plants during the conversion of glucose and is believed to attack the nucleophilic centres of the bacterial cell's DNA molecule. This renders the cell unable to produce new proteins and contributes to a breakdown of the cell.

Methyl-glyoxal content

Methyl-glyoxal (MG) in manuka honey has been shown to originate from di-hydroxy-acetone (DHA), present in varying amounts, in the nectar of manuka flowers. Freshly produced manuka honey contains low levels of MG and high levels of DHA. Researchers found that storage of these honeys at 37°C led to a decrease in the DHA content and a related increase in methyl-glyoxal. Very low, but measurable, levels of MG, sometimes written as MGO, are found in most honeys. Manuka honey has been shown to have levels several hundred times greater.

The 2006 German discovery, with research[14] published in 2008, showed that naturally occurring methyl-glyoxal is the dominant constituent in manuka honey, responsible for much of its antibacterial properties. MG levels in manuka honey varied from 30 mg per kg to 700 mg per kg. A minimum MG level of 100 mg per kg was needed in order to effectively inhibit the growth of *Staphylococcus aureus*.

Further, there was an indication that the UMF-value, the commercially used parameter to rate the antibacterial activity of manuka honey, is directly related to the content of MGO. It was unambiguously demonstrated for the first time that MGO is directly responsible for the antibacterial activity

Plate 1: Chapter 5 Microbiology Explained

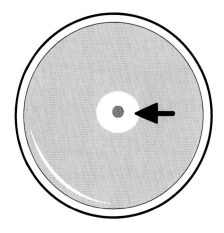

Fig 2. Zone of Inhibition of bacterial growth indicates
activity of antimicrobial product.

Plate 2: Chapter 5 Microbiology Explained

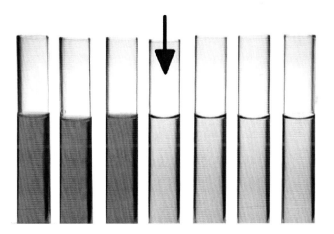

Fig. 3 The first tube where there is no growth
(indicated by the arrow) is the MIC.

Plate 3: Chapter 5 Microbiology Explained

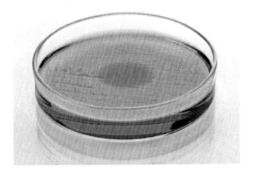

Fig. 4 Zone of Inhibition plate. The cleared central area is where the essential oil has destroyed the bacteria.

Plate 4: Chapter 8 Thyme

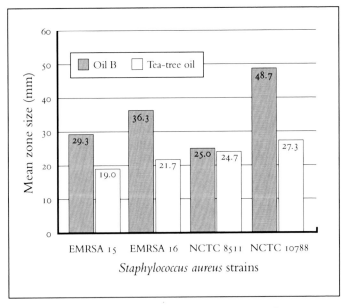

Fig. 1 Bar chart comparing tea tree to Oil B.

Plate 5: Chapter 8 Thyme

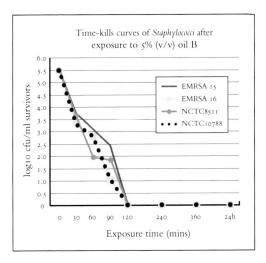

Fig. 2 Time-kill curves for Oil B thyme blend.

Plate 6: Chapter 8 Thyme

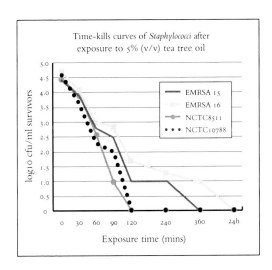

Fig. 3 Time-kill curves for tea tree.

PLATE 7

Plate 7: Chapter 8 Thyme

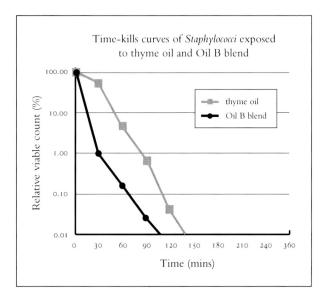

Fig. 4 Time-kill curves for all staphylococci exposed
to thyme oil and Oil B blend.

of manuka honey, but the story is not yet fully told. As Professor Henle's paper states: "at present, only speculations can be made concerning the origin of MGO in manuka honey."

The paper concluded: "with the present investigation, the occurrence of high amounts of MGO in New Zealand manuka honey was demonstrated. MGO was identified as a bioactive compound responsible for the antibacterial activity of these honey samples. Studies in order to clarify the pathways for the biochemical formation of MGO in manuka plants and honey are underway in our laboratory."

UMF and MG/MGO

In regards to the antibacterial rating system for manuka honey the consensus seems to be:

- **Methyl-glyoxal** is responsible for the antibacterial activity of manuka honey and equates to the Unique Manuka Factor (the non-peroxide antibacterial activity).

- **UMF** equates to the antibacterial power of phenol dilutions with UMF 10 being equal to a 10% phenol solution.

- **Methyl-glyoxal** is measured in grams:
  MG 100 or **MGO 100** = 100grams methyl-glyoxal in 1 kilo honey.

- **UMF 10** is comparable to **MGO 100**.

A minimum level of MGO 100 or UMF 10 is needed to inhibit the growth of *Staphylococcus aureus*, and because there is a different rating system for MGO and UMF it could be a little confusing, as the following demonstrates:

- UMF 20 is twice as potent as UMF 10.

- But: MGO 400 is twice as potent as MGO 100.

- So: UMF 10 = MGO 100 and UMF 20 = MGO 400.

See *Resources: Manuka Honey,* for information on ratings.

Further research, into the detection and measurement of methyl-glyoxal, has taken place in New Zealand[15] with several papers and articles being published. Ongoing university research in both hemispheres of the world is trying to come to a definitive conclusion as to why the nectar of manuka flowers creates an antibacterial honey.

Relationship of plant, essential oil and honey

In 2007, a team of researchers[16] in New Zealand obtained dozens of honey samples in order to identify variations in methyl-glyoxal levels and to try to find out why the variations occurred. They did this by isolating different fractions of manuka honey and analysing each component by High Performance Liquid Chromatography (HPLC) and concluded: "methyl-glyoxal levels in some plants increase significantly, from two to six fold, in response to salinity, drought and cold stress. Much of the manuka honey comes from areas deemed too marginal for farming. It is possible that the soil and climatic conditions in these areas are contributing high stress levels to the plant. The excess methyl-glyoxal produced is then transferred to the honey."

According to a 2008 article in New Zealand Beekeeper[17], Professor Molan and his team analysed manuka honey and essential oil of manuka profiles and had this to say: "… tree populations in Central North Island and East Coast represented *Leptospermum scoparium* var. *myrtifolium* and an unnamed variety of manuka. The latter, growing principally on the East coast, contains triketones in the essential oil, giving the oil antibacterial activity."

The 2009,[15] New Zealand research looking for the origin of methylglyoxal in manuka honey said: "we conclude that the methylglyoxal in NZ manuka honey is derived by the non-enzymatic conversion of di-hydroxyacetone which occurs at high levels in the nectar for reasons which are as yet unknown." When looking at the various regional manuka honeys, Molan's team found that different varieties of *Leptospermum scoparium* in diverse areas of the North and South Island contributed to the various UMF levels. The research also uncovered that nectar from plants other than the manuka plant could be a significant ingredient in some manuka honey and that this fact would influence the UMF ratings.

At the present time there is evidence to suggest that the aroma-chemistry of manuka plants is ultimately responsible for the antibacterial activity of manuka honey, but in scientific terms, there is as yet, insufficient evidence to make such a statement.

Microbiology research with manuka honey

In 1991, after intensive research that looked at different levels of the antibacterial effects of honey, Waikato University published a paper[18] on the antibacterial activity of some New Zealand honeys. Years of laboratory research then went into confirming that manuka honey was most suited to killing *Staphylococcus aureus*, a Gram-positive bacteria. *Staph aureus* is mankind's most common bacteria but as it has developed resistance to many antibiotics commonly used in hospitals, it has become the predominant cause of wound sepsis. This is why the main focus of research with manuka honey has been with *Staph aureus* and MRSA. Although the antibacterial potency of honey is insufficient to allow its use systemically, there are various clinical applications besides wound care in which it is used topically. The Waikato University has a Honey Research Unit which is engaged in ongoing research with manuka honey.

In the United Kingdom, doctors at The Christie, a Manchester hospital, have been involved with a small clinical trial studying the use of manuka honey in patients with cancer of the mouth and throat, in order to reduce their risk of becoming infected with MRSA. *In vitro* tests are generally followed by animal testing before progressing to clinical trials. As medical grade manuka honey works in a gentle way, and is also a food, there has been no need for animal testing and clinical trials have already begun.

In 2008, researchers[19] undertook a systematic review of other previously published research papers into the use of manuka (and other honey) in preventing MRSA infection in oncology patients. They concluded that "honey was found to be a suitable alternative for wound healing, burns and various skin conditions, and to potentially have a role within cancer care."

Researchers[20] at the University of Wales in 2009, conducted research with three commercially available wound dressings, each impregnated with manuka honey. Epidemic strain EMRS-15 was the bacteria used across all test materials. Results showed that all three products had an ability to kill off the bacteria. At the end of six hours, two had reduced the bacteria to negligable levels. The third reduced the bacterial load by a smaller amount within the same timeframe.

Medical grade manuka honey

In order for a manuka honey to achieve the status of a medicinal honey and be used in wound dressings, it must hold the European Conformity (CE) mark and have regulatory approval as a sterile Medical Device. Medical grade manuka honey products are gaining acceptance in hospitals and clinics for the treatment of wounds, burns and skin ulcers. There is a reduction in inflammation, and both swelling and pain are reduced. Infected wounds give off a bad odour which is eliminated by the regular use of manuka products. The consistancy and properties of manuka honey make it easier for wounds to heal. Dead tissue is drawn into the honey, and because honey always retains its moisture, this facilitates the painless removal of dressings without damaging new skin tissue. This results in quicker healing, less scarring and significantly less distress for the patient when dressings are changed.

Several companies are now producing manuka impregnated wound dressings as well as creams for topical application. Excellent results are being obtained on infected wounds which were not responding to standard antibiotic and antiseptic therapy. Reports from medical personnel already utilising manuka honey in a hospital environment are that UMF10 is adequate for treating leg ulcers, but to treat serious bacterial infection it is recommended to use UMF15 or higher. Manuka honey with a quality assured level of antibacterial activity is used by the companies marketing manuka honey products for wound care. Every product has to conform to strict guidelines set down by the European regulatory agencies.

Contra-indications

Manuka honey and products containing manuka honey should not be used by:

- Anyone with a known sensitivity to bees.

- Babies under the age of 1 year: honey sometimes contains spores of *Clostridium botulinum.*

- Some hayfever sufferers.

- Vegans: as honey is produced by hard working bees and is the hive's winter foodstore.

- Diabetics are advised to not consume manuka honey, although it is safe to treat a wound with a manuka honey wound dressing, as the sugars in honey cannot be absorbed through the skin. However, a diabetic person with a wound should in the first instance seek medical attention.

Chapter 8

Thyme

Thousands of tons of thyme are harvested annually, much of which is dried and sold as a food condiment. It is a familiar herb for kitchen use and an important component of 'bouquet garni'. Thyme oil, the essential oil distilled from the herb, is classed as one of the world's top ten essential oils because of its wide variety of applications. Thyme is a low-lying shrub that generally grows no higher than 50 cm, although some species can grow up to a metre tall. A minority of thymes, such as *Thymus serpyllum* (wild thyme) are creeping plants, lacking the woody stems of most other thymes. All thyme plants flower according to season and location. Flowers can be white, pink or purple. There are an estimated 350 species of thyme growing in the world, many with subspecies, but only a handful grown commercially – mostly in Spain Portugal and France. There is also a market for wild crafted (collected by hand) thymes in a dozen or so countries.

Thyme *(Thymus)*
Common thymes are *Thymus vulgaris* and *Thymus zygis*.

Geographical location: Thyme is thought to have originated in the Western Mediterranean region but it extends eastwards in Asia, up to the Himalayas, to China and Japan. It can be found along the north coast of Africa and on the Sinai Peninsula. The herb has been introduced to countries as far south and east as Chile and New Zealand, and north and westwards to the UK, Germany, Poland, Bulgaria, Hungary, Russia and Canada. In general thyme is a sun-loving plant, although some species can live in very cold climates, such as Siberia and Greenland.

Habitat and how it alters the chemistry
The thyme plant is polymorphous. Polymorphism means that within the plant chemical changes occur, many times over, depending on the environment in which it is growing. So, for example, if several identical common thyme

plants (*Thymus vulgaris*) were to be planted in different locations and altitudes, and furthermore, that each was subject to differing soil types, levels of sunshine, exposure to or protection from wind and early morning frosts, then the individual thymes would vary in their mix of aroma chemicals. Researchers[1] in the south of France carried out such an experiment in and around a valley. The results of chemical analysis demonstrated the thyme plant's ability for adaptive variation. Charles Darwin first noted this process of natural selection among thyme plants. Some of the numerous *Thymus vulgaris* sub-species have been deliberately cloned in order to produce a plant with a specific chemotype. For example, a plant rich in thymol will be of significant importance to some, whereas a thyme rich in linalool may be of great interest to others. Thyme oil is universally recognized as being one of the most powerful of aromatic plants. Authors of books promoting the use of essential oils, advise caution when using thyme oil. It is useful to have some comprehension of thyme's polymorphous qualities, as it goes some way towards explaining why some thymes are too powerful to use on the skin of healthy adults whilst other thymes can be safely used on children.

Thyme products

The cultivation of thyme is split between the fresh herb for culinary use, the whole plant for garden use, the dried herb for culinary/food industry use, the dried herb from which a tincture is obtained for medicinal use and the essential oil which is mainly sold to the food industry, but increasingly to the pharmaceutical, aromatherapy and natural cosmetics industries.

Thyme oil from Spain is usually red when distilled, and is sold as 'red thyme'. The red colour is caused by a reaction between the thymol content of the plant and the iron in the field stills. 'White thyme' is not a separate species of thyme, but is rectified red thyme oil. What this means is that the red thyme oil is distilled for a second time in stainless steel equipment. White thyme has a high thymol content as the rectification process causes a loss of some of the more volatile aromatic compounds.

Thyme essential oil

Of the variety of thymes under cultivation for their essential oil, the five species of greatest economic importance are: *Thymus vulgaris, Thymus zygis, Thymus capitatus, Thymus serpyllum* and *Thymus mastichina*. Of the aroma chemicals found within the plants, the most widely used compounds are thymol and carvacrol, followed by linalool. Both thymol and carvacrol are phenols, which can be irritating to the skin. For this reason some thyme growers have sought to clone the linalool and geraniol chemotypes for the aromatherapy and toiletries market, as the phenol content of these chemotypes is greatly reduced. Thymes with high levels of thymol and carvacrol have been found to be the most antimicrobial and are used in the food industry to extend the shelf life of meats and processed food. Thyme essential oil and thymol are acquired by the pharmaceutical industry for use in cough medicines and for oral hygiene products.

Commercially available thyme oil is generally labelled as 'red thyme' or 'white thyme'. Red thyme oil is the crude product of common thyme, whereas white thyme oil, as mentioned, is rectified red thyme.

The Chemistry of Thyme

Within thyme plants there are dozens of different aromatic compounds. The twenty most common are listed in order of the quantity obtained:

1. Thymol	8. Geraniol	15. Citral
2. Carvacrol	9. Alpha-terpinene	16. Myrcene
3. Linalool	10. Alpha-terpineol	17. Terpinen-4-ol
4. Para-cymene	11. Beta-caryophyllene	18. Trans-sabinene
5. Gamma-terpinene	12. Geranyl acetate	19. Alpha-pinene
6. Borneol	13. Camphor	20. Camphene
7. 1,8-cineole	14. Linalyl acetate	+ Minor constituents*

*added together contribute to a small percentage of the entire oil

Typical chemistry of common thyme (*Thymus vulgaris*)

Phenols:	Thymol 66.95% + carvacrol 3.73	= 70.73%
Alcohols:	Linalool 2.51% + terpinen-4-ol 0.72%	= 3.23%
Terpenes:	Total combined terpenes*	= 20.49%

*Para-cymene 10.83%, gamma-terpinene 5.23%, alpha-pinene 0.43%, camphene 0.22%, myrcene 0.84%, alpha-terpinene 0.69, limonene 0.35%, beta-caryophyllene 1.9%

Scientific research with thyme oil

Thyme oil has been used as a fumigant in sick rooms and places of worship by many ancient civilizations. As far back as 1887[2], thyme was recognized as having antibacterial properties, although it wasn't until the 1980s that it became the subject of scientific interest. The majority of microbiology research into thyme's ability to kill bacteria has been published in food journals. Thyme oil, along with some other essential oils, is widely recognized as a reliable preservative for the food industry.

Another strand of research has been with the plaque-inhibiting properties of thyme oil and thymol (the plant's major constituent) which has led to thyme oil being widely used as a treatment for, and deterrent against, gum disease. It is found in over-the-counter oral hygiene products. However, the use of thyme in the pharmaceutical industry has remained small in comparison to its use in the food industry.

There has been little enthusiasm for the employment of thyme for topical use as the chemical makeup of most thymes contain significant levels of phenols, which can be an irritant to the skin. Many species of thyme contain in excess of 50% phenols (a combination of thymol and carvacrol), with some thymes containing 80% phenols. In the 1990s, researchers[3] established that thymol and carvacrol were effective against plaque, a biofilm affecting the teeth. Subsequent research looked at several essential oils, including common thyme, for their *in vitro* activity against antibiotic resistant organisms. One of the many bacteria responsible for food decay is *Staphylococcus aureus*; so it is the common *staph* bacterium, and not MRSA, which has been the subject of most of the microbiology research with thyme oil.

In 1993, *Thymus vulgaris* was one of the eleven aromatic plants tested against twenty five test organisms by an Italian research cohort[4]. All the aromatic plants were growing in Northern Italy. The strain of *Staph aureus* tested was not specified: "all the essential oils from the plants studied possessed main components that were found to be biologically active, namely thymol, carvacrol, p–cymene, gamma–terpinene, 1,8–cineole, cis–ocimene, camphor, linalool, terpinen-4-ol, thujone, limonene, alpha–bisabol and chamazulene." They concluded: "it is not possible to establish a relationship between oil composition and biological activity due to the synergistic action between certain components."

In 1998, a patent[5] was filed for a Broad Spectrum Antibiotic. It consisted of a mixture of tea tree and thyme oils. The specific thymes used in this research were White thyme (rectified *Thymus vulgaris*) and Wild thyme, (*Thymus serpyllum*). *Staph aureus* was tested but the actual strain was not specified. Zones of inhibition, called 'halos' in the patent application, were measured with the following results:

Tea tree = 10 mm

Thyme = 18 mm

Mixture of tea tree and thyme = 26 mm.

The patent application was withdrawn in 2000.

Italian researchers[6] looked at the antimicrobial capabilities of four thymes: three growing in Sardinia and one commercially purchased. When the chemistry of each oil was analysed, the phenolic compounds thymol and carvacrol constituted the major constituents of each oil, with phenol quantities of 48.9%, 40.1%, 53.1%, and 67.5%. The linalool content ranged from 3.3% to 10.3%. The terpinen-4-ol levels were 0% to 1%. The *Staph aureus* strains were mainly taken from rotting food. Also included was a reference stock of *Staph* ATCC 25923. "Generally, the oils exhibited similar (to each other) levels of antimicrobial activity, but one of the thymes appeared to be more efficient … in particular against *Staph aureus* and four other bacteria." This thyme oil contained the highest concentrations of phenols, at 67.5%.

In 2007, researchers[7] in Spain looked at three species of thyme (some with chemotypes) growing in Murcia, as antimicrobial agents for the food industry. There are ten microorganisms of significant importance in the food industry and each was assessed against the thyme oils. The strain of *Staph aureus* tested was CECT 239.

Results against *Staph aureus*	Total phenols	ZOI
Thymus zygis		
Chemotype – thymol	71.6%	25.0 mm
Chemotype – 39% linalool	0.5%	18.3 mm
Chemotype – 82% linalool	2.2%	18.6 mm

Thymus vulgaris

Chemotype – thymol	61.8%	45.0 mm

Thymus hyemalis

Chemotype – carvacrol	48.4%	35.0 mm
Chemotype – thymol/linalool	18.0%	32.3 mm
Chemotype – thymol	43.9%	38.6 mm

MIC and MBC tests showed that the most antimicrobial thymes were *T. hyemalis* (thymol and carvacrol chemotypes), *T. zygis* (thymol chemotype) and *T. vulgaris* (thymol chemotype).

"In our study, most of the antimicrobial activity in essential oils from the thymus genus appears to be associated with the phenolic compounds: thymol and carvacrol." However the authors concluded that minor compounds could play an important part in the antimicrobial potency of the oil:"results suggest that it could be a synergistic action among phenolic compounds and cited compounds."

Canadian researchers[8] evaluated twenty-eight essential oils for their antibacterial properties against four bacteria prevalent in the food industry. *Staphylococcus aureus* was one of the four. Of the essential oils tested, the most effective were thyme oils. *Thymus vulgaris* (chemotype thymol), *Thymus serpyllum*, and *Thymus satureiodes*, each having significant levels of thymol and carvacrol, were found to be the most effective against the four bacterial pathogens responsible for outbreaks of food poisoning. Other varieties of thyme: *Thymus mastichina*, *Thymus vulgaris* (chemotype thuyanol), *Thymus vulgaris* (chemotype linalool), were still effective but required a higher dosage to inhibit bacterial growth. The most effective essential oil was a close relative of thyme, Spanish oregano (*Thymus capitatus*), containing 76% carvacrol and 5% thymol. In Canada alone, the cost of treating foodborne disease due to contamination with bacteria is estimated to be $500 million a year.

The above results bear out those of numerous other researchers: that thyme oils with high levels of phenols are very effective agents against *Staphylococcus aureus* and other bacteria, and are perfectly suited for use in the food industry.

Very little research has been carried out into the bacteriostatic properties of thyme oil against MRSA. There is some published MRSA research that includes mention of white thyme oil being used in tandem with manufactured antimicrobials such as quaternary ammonium.

In 1997, research[9] compared the efficacy of thyme oil against the essential oils of tea tree, lavender, mint, and juniper, after each had been challenged with fifteen strains of MRSA isolates taken from hospital in-patients. Results showed that tea tree was the most bactericidal / bacteriostatic. "Tea tree oil was the most potent of the five oils ... these results are identical to those reported previously for strains isolated in both the UK and Australia."

In laboratory studies, US researchers[10] compared three different pharmaceutical compounds against four strains of MRSA. The compounds were: neomycin + polymyxin, polymyxin + gramicidin, benzethonium chloride (a quaternary ammonium) + tea tree + white thyme oil. This last blend had the most rapid action.

To sum up: out of several hundred species of thyme, only a few have been used in microbiology research, and often without an analysis of the oil's chemistry. Primarily the research has centred on common thyme, and its major compounds, as a food preservative. To date, when thyme has been used in MRSA research, it has either been in combination with other antimicrobials or, when it comes under comparison with other essential oils, it has been found to be less effective than tea tree oil.

Thyme vs MRSA: new microbiology research

In 2003, I began my own studies into MRSA. I was looking for an essential oil, or blend of essential oils, powerful enough to kill the evolving superbug. I had already studied and written about tea tree oil and was impressed with its pedigree. However, as two of my three children are unable to tolerate tea tree oil on their skin, and a small percentage of users, worldwide, are estimated to have experienced similar problems, I was hoping to find a viable alternative. In 2005, I began working with scientists at the University of Brighton[11] to try to find an effective essential oil, or blend of essential oils, that would be safe to use whilst having the ability to kill epidemic strains EMRSA-15 and EMRSA-16. Common thyme oil was not included in tests, as its skin irritant factor is well known, but I did include a sub species of thyme – a thyme linalool – which produced good results against both epidemic strains as well as two strains of MSSA (methicillin sensitive *Staphylococcus aureus*).

A search was then made to find a consistently available source of the right sort of thyme oil, as without a secure supply chain the research would remain academic. Eventually I began working with a distiller of essential oils with a vast knowledge of essential oil chemistry, in order to find the perfect combination of thyme oils. Several different thymes were investigated, resulting in a blend of four thymes which gave a thyme linalool with a slightly higher thymol content than is normally found in a thyme linalool. With a further round of university microbiology tests already scheduled, I sent through the thyme blend, which became known as 'Oil B' in testing. This round of tests challenged epidemic strains EMRSA-15 and EMRSA-16, and two MSSA with three different tea tree oils as well as Oil B, and a comparison of the results was made.

The outcome of the research was better than expected. The original thyme sub – species had a predominant linalool content with a small percentage of thymol and carvacrol. Oil B had roughly equal proportions of linalool and thymol, and there was a very exciting discovery: Oil B also contained significant levels of terpinen-4-ol, common in tea tree oil, but

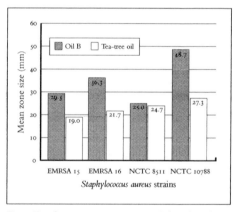

Fig. 1   Bar chart comparing tea tree to Oil B (see Plate 4).

which does not often appear in thyme oils. The thyme oil blend had a unique combination of major compounds and was effective at killing epidemic strains EMRSA-15 and EMRSA-16 using a 5% dilution.

Typical chemistry of thyme linalool

Linalool   11% – 60%

Thymol   1.3% – 15%

Oil B is approximately 24% linalool 31% thymol. At approximately 11% terpinen-4-ol is also a significant component.

The combination of aroma chemistry: roughly equal proportions of phenols + alcohols + terpenes, was found to completely eradicate epidemic strains EMRSA-15 and EMRSA-16 within a period of two hours. These results were compared to the kill rate for tea tree against the same bacterial strains. See Figs. 2 and 3 for comparison.

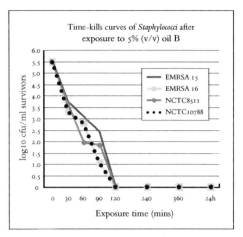

Fig. 2 Time-kill curves for Oil B thyme blend (see Plate 5).

Tea tree has long been thought of as the benchmark by which to measure the efficacy of other essential oils when looking to find a natural antibacterial. So when it was found that Oil B was equal to, and sometimes significantly better than, tea tree oil, Oil B became known as Benchmark thyme. After the university microbiology trials with tea tree had been completed, a further round of research[12] took place: challenging Oil B and the

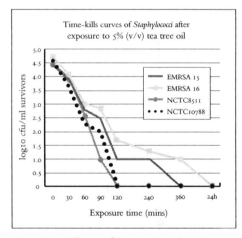

Fig. 3 Time-kill curves for tea tree (see Plate 6).

original thyme linalool sample with the two MSSA strains and the epidemic strains EMRSA-15 and EMRSA-16. Both oils worked effectively against the four test bacteria but in kill curves it was seen that Oil B worked faster, and in zone of inhibition tests it was Oil B that produced the largest zones. Growth controls showed an increase in bacterial numbers to be between log 2 and log 3 by the end of six hours. Both the thymes caused a log 2 – log 3 reduction in all four bacterial strains within three hours. The single thyme linalool took two and a half hours to reduce the numbers to zero whereas Oil B reduced bacterial numbers to zero within two hours. In both cases, a 3 log decrease in bacterial numbers was observed, indicating a strong bactericidal effect.

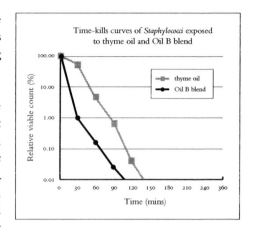

Of the 350 species of thyme in the world, the most researched to date have been the common thyme: *Thymus vulgaris* and *Thymus zygis*. The University of Brighton research has produced interesting results using lesser known thyme oils against multi-drug resistant bacteria.

Fig. 4 Time-kill curves for all staphylococci exposed to thyme oil and Oil B blend (see Plate 7).

With hundreds of other thyme oils not yet investigated, the potential exists for further breakthroughs in the fight against microbial evolution. Although clinical trials would be needed to substantiate the effectiveness of these products in the treatment of MRSA colonised or infected wounds, microbiology results demonstrate the ability of some types of thyme oil to kill MRSA *in vitro*.

Contra-indications

- Thyme oils can be used in the treatment of dogs and horses with appropriate advice.

- Cats cannot metabolise phenols, so thyme must never be used for the treatment of a cat.

- As all thyme oils are irritant to mucous membranes, they are not ideally suited for nasal decolonisation as they will recreate the symptoms of a cold.

- If any skin irritation is experienced then cease use and find alternative essential oils.

Chapter 9

Further Research with Essential Oils

Essential oils have a long history of use in combating infection and many are marketed for their antiseptic properties. Science is now backing up these claims and an internet search for 'antimicrobial research with essential oils' will bring up hundreds of research papers. Scientific research is ongoing, and as recently as November 2010, an international conference on antimicrobial research took place in Spain.[1] One session, entitled: "Antimicrobial natural products", covered a wide range of natural substances, essential oils and aromatic plants, and examples from each category were among the many subjects under review.

Presentations included research papers on the following: geraniol (from geranium oil), a compound found to restore activities against multidrugresistant isolates from Gram-negative species; curcumin, from cumin seeds, as a potential natural antibiofilm agent; bactericidal activity of essential oil of *Cymbopogon citratus* (lemongrass); and antimicrobial activity of essential oil extracts on bacterial isolates from the blood stream of HIV infected patients.

There is no shortage of academic evidence to show that essential oils and their individual components are antimicrobial, but having access to the research is just the first step on a long flight of stairs. Unfortunately, each ascending step has onerous costs and difficulties, mainly with the setting up of clinical trials and the gaining of regulatory approval that only large, financially strong companies can consider undertaking. This chapter covers a selection of the work carried out in laboratories around the world, mostly looking at bacteriostatic activity against *Staph aureus*, whilst others focus on bactericidal activity against MRSA.

Lelechwa

Lelechwa, sometimes spelled leleshwa, came to the attention of an observant woman[2] living in Kenya, when, during wildlife protection operations in the 1980s, it was first noticed that the black rhino being fitted with a radio transmitter had an unblemished skin, even though it was a mature male. Subsequently it was noted that other animals frequenting the lelechwa groves and rubbing against the aromatic leaves had skin that was free from the usual infected scratches, septic wounds, fungal infections and parasites common in wild animals elsewhere in Kenya. It was this observation that lead to the plant being distilled and analysed.

Lelechwa (*Tarchonanthus camphorates*)

Also known as African Wild Sage and Camphor Bush. It has many African dialect names.

Geographical location: The Great Rift Valley, Kenya. The plant grows naturally all along the Great Rift Valley into east and southern Africa.

Habitat

Lelechwa grows to a height of ten to eighteen feet, in poor soil, on the highlands of the Kenyan Great Rift Valley, and is suited to the prevailing dry conditions of the area. Thick groves of lelechwa provide shelter for large animals such as rhino, elephants and buffalo. As lelechwa is inedible and has no natural pests, it has grown freely and extensively and was, until recently, thought to be a weed as it was practically impossible to destroy.

The plant and products

Most parts of the plant are usable. The dried roots are suitable for carvings, the stems turned into slow burning 'eco-charcoal' and the leaves are distilled to produce an essential oil. Nothing much was known about the aromatic leaves other than, since time immemorial, the plant had been used by the Maasai as a natural deodorant, and that the plant and its essential oil act as a natural insect repellent. Today, a toiletries product range[3] with medicinal properties based on lelechwa has been developed in Africa. The first prototype still for steam distillation of lelechwa leaves was installed in 1989. Subsequent UK analysis[4] found that lelechwa was highly antiseptic with additional antifungal and insect repellent properties. The essential oil is a pale yellow/green colour, with a camphor-like, almost medicinal aroma.

Chemistry

When analysed by gas chromatography-mass spectrometry, lelechwa was identified as being composed of:

fenchol	15.9%	1,8-cineol	14.3%
eucalyptol	13.9%	alpha-terpineol	13.2%
alpha-pinene	6.87%	trans-pinene hydrate	6.51%
terpinen-4-ol	4.74%	camphene	3.76%

+beta-pinene, delta-2-carene, alpha-phellandrene, limonene, gamma-terpinene, terpinolene, fenchone, trans-caryophyllene, bergamotene, delta-cadinene and alpha-curcumene.

Microbiology

Microbiology research has been undertaken in order to support a patent[5] application for the use of lelechwa in medicated products, with its use against MRSA being one of the main 'inventions'. One of the claims is that: "compositions of the invention can be used... in the control of airborne infection and for routine protection against antibiotic resistant bacteria such as, for example, MRSA."

In 2005, an international team of scientists[6] conducted microbiological tests with lelechwa against a range of microoganisms. The essential oil was screened for antimicrobial activity against both Gram-positive (which included *Stapylococcus aureus*) and Gram-negative bacteria, as well as a pathogenic fungus. With the exception of one of the Gram-negatives that showed resistance, lelechwa oil had pronounced antibacterial and antifungal activities.

Agonis

Agonis fragrans is a fairly new essential oil to the commercial market in comparison to tea tree and eucalyptus oils which have been exported from Australia for decades. Research into the uses of agonis is in its infancy; it belongs to the *Myrtacaea* family along with tea tree, eucalyptus, manuka and myrtle. This shrub has undergone a few name changes[7] in just over a decade. Since 1998, it has been known as *Agonis* sp. coarse tea tree, *Agonis* sp. Coarse *Agonis* and *Agonis fragrans* but since 2007 it has been called

Taxandria fragrans by Western Australian Flora, although *Agonis fragrans* is still in use. It is sometimes referred to as Fragrant Ti-tree.

Agonis (*Taxandria fragrans*)

Geographical location: The agonis tree is native to the south-west corner of Western Australia, but is now being grown commercially across Western Australia, notably between Perth and Albany.

Habitat

The shrub grows up to two metres tall and flowers between February and May. The flowers are clustered toward the end of stems/branches and resemble manuka flowers with small white petals surrounding a dark red centre. It likes waterlogged soil and can be found in swampy areas and along waterways. The distilled oil is pale yellow. The aroma is described variously as: citrusy, spicy-cinnamon, and sweet balsamic.

Commercial production of agonis began in the 1990s, with establishment of plantations in the south western corner of Western Australia.[8] A particular clone is now being marketed internationally for the treatment of minor ailments and for use in cosmetic products.

Chemistry

Analysis[9] of the high cineol agonis shows the proportion of aroma-chemicals across five essential oil samples to be between:

1,8-cineole	28.3 - 34.1%	alpha-pinene	13.7 - 28.0%
linalool	3.3 - 14.7%	alpha-terpineol	5.2 - 5.9%
myrtenol	1.7 - 5.5%	terpinen-4-ol	2.9 - 3.9%
para-cymene	2.4 - 2.8%	myrcene	1.6 - 2.7%
gamma-terpinene	1.9 - 2.4%	beta pinene	1.4 - 1.9%

+ minor aroma-chemicals across all five oils tested, ranged from 0-3.8%

Less common than the high cineole agonis is the low-cineole variant, which when analysed shows a breakdown of:

alpha-pinene	1.5%	linalool	25.3%
myrtenol	20.0%	1,8-cineole	1.0%

Microbiology

A group of Australian researchers[10] in 2007/2008, were asked to investigate the potential antibacterial activity of the essential oil distilled from a selection of agonis plants. A wide variety of clinical isolates and reference strains were obtained from Australian laboratories.[11] Those selected were a broad range of Gram-positive and Gram-negative bacteria and some yeasts. The *Staph aureus* chosen was *Staphylococcus aureus* NCTC 6571 along with other variants of *staphylococcus*. All five of the agonis samples exhibited significant inhibitory activity against the selected strains, with minor differences between the sample oils. Time-kill curves showed a greater than log 3 reduction in two hours for two of the five sample oils when tested against *Staphylococcus aureus* 6571. The *staph* had not been completely eradicated within 2 hours and the data does not show what length of time would be necessary to effect a complete kill. However the data does support the anti-inflammatory properties of agonis, which could be useful in addressing the inflammatory response to infection.

Essential oils and blends vs MRSA for the treatment of burns

Many essential oils have antibacterial properties, but when it comes to killing *Staph aureus* and MRSA bacteria, a successful outcome is not guaranteed. In 2004, a team of UK researchers[12] set up microbiology tests to determine whether blends of essential oils could work more effectively than single essential oils.

The essential oils under trial were:

• Tea tree (*Melaleuca alternifolia*)

• Geranium (*Pelargonium graveolens*)

• Lavender (*Lavandula angustfolia*)

• Patchouli (*Pogostemon cablin*)

Tests involved putting the essential oils directly onto paper discs that were then placed on agar plates containing the bacterial growth. The strains used for the research were: antibiotic susceptible strain *Staphylococcus aureus* NCTC 6571 (Oxford strain), two MRSA samples obtained from the wounds of a burns patient: an untyped MRSA strain and the epidemic strain EMRSA-15.

Some inhibition was seen with each essential oil whether single or combined with another oil. When used singly, tea tree was the most effective at inhibiting growth of MRSA bacteria. Interestingly, when tea tree was included in a blend with other essential oils, the susceptibility of *Staph aureus* 6571 increased, but against MRSA strains the effect decreased.

A commercially available grapefruit seed extract[13] was added to each essential oil and further tests took place, showing that some combinations were more effective than the single oil and some were less so. Effectiveness was more prominent in tests with *Staph aureus* 6571 whilst other tests showed increased inhibition with MRSA strains.

Overall, the best results against MRSA were obtained with tea tree on its own although there was antimicrobial activity when tea tree was used in combination with lavender or grapefruit seed extract. With both contact and vapour diffusion, the oil blends had greater effect than the individual essential oils. When a commercial burn dressing was used in combination with essential oils/essential oil blends, results were varied but overall the inhibitory action was good. The degree of inhibition depended on the brand of dressing.[14]

Vapour testing

Vapour testing of single and combined essential oils was also investigated. One of the most noticeable things about essential oils is their aroma. The vapours released from essential oils have been proven to be highly antimicrobial. The most efficient system of diffusing essential oils into the air is with the use of 'Venturi technology'.[15] A suitable machine[16] was used, where air is forced over the surface of an essential oil, or essential oil blend, allowing the antimicrobial vapours to be released into the atmosphere. Testing showed that the single oils produced little or no inhibition of the bacteria, whereas some of the combinations had good zones of inhibition. The research paper[17] concluded: "Essential oils have a huge potential for exploitation in the healthcare setting over the forthcoming years. Many of the bacteria we now see routinely in hospitals are resistant to most antibiotics and alternative treatments have to be found. Essential oils offer a whole new concept to prevention and treatment of infectious disease in the future."

More research with antimicrobial essential oils

United States
Utah
Research conducted in 2008, at a Utah university,[18] looked at the inhibitory effects of ninety one single essential oils and sixty four blends of essential oils on the growth of *Staphylococcus aureus*. The bacterium used was an MRSA staph ATCC 700699[19] tested on agar plates at a non-specified inoculum.

Of the ninety-one single oils tested, the zone of inhibition results demonstrated that the majority had inhibitory properties. The essential oils with a zone of inhibition of 50 mm or larger were: lemon myrtle, lemongrass, melissa, mountain savoury, cinnamon bark, cumin, lemon scented eucalyptus and common thyme. Of the blends, a handful had inhibition zones of 50 mm or more. Zone of inhibition tests are used for first stage research to ascertain the minimum inhibitory concentration.

United Kingdom
Ayrshire
The antimicrobial activity of a selection of essential oils was investigated in a Scottish college[20] in 1999. The essential oils under consideration were: black pepper, clove, geranium, nutmeg, oregano and common thyme. Each oil was tested against twenty-five bacteria, which included *Staph aureus*. Components with the widest spectrum of activity were found to be, in descending order: thymol, carvacrol, alpha-terpineol, terpinen-4-ol, eugenol, linalool, followed by the components exhibiting lesser activity.

The researchers found: "the volatile oils exhibited considerable inhibitory effects against all the organisms under test while their major components demonstrated various degrees of growth inhibition" and concluded, "the plant extracts clearly demonstrate antibacterial properties, although the mechanistic processes are poorly understood. These activities suggest potential use as chemotherapeutic agents, food preserving agents and disinfectants. Their volatility would be a distinct advantage in lowering microbial contamination in air and on difficult to reach surfaces."

India
Bhubaneswar
India is a country where aromatic plants grow in abundance. Many are commercially grown, not only for food spices, but also for their essential

oils. Researchers[21] in India looked into the antimicrobial properties of ten essential oils, two of them not widely available. Of the eight oils of general interest, each was tested for antibacterial activity against twentytwo bacteria, which included *Staphylococcus aureus*. The essential oils were: citronella, eucalyptus, geranium, lemongrass, orange, palmarosa, patchouli and peppermint.

The overall inhibitory results were as follows: lemongrass, eucalyptus, peppermint and orange oils were effective against all the twenty-two bacterial strains. Palmarosa oil inhibited twenty-one bacteria, patchouli inhibited twenty, citronella fifteen strains and geranium oil was inhibitory to twelve bacterial strains. The MIC of the oils varied widely, with some essential oils working at very low dilution and others requiring a more than a hundred fold stronger dilution before they were effective at inhibiting growth of the bacteria.

Chennai
To evaluate the antibacterial activity of twenty-one plant essential oils against six bacterial species, a team of microbiologists[22] in Chennai set up a research programme. Six microorganisms were obtained[23] which included *Staphylococcus aureus* ATCC 25923. The objective was to determine the minimum levels of each essential oil needed in order to prevent growth of bacterial culture.

Results revealed that the selected essential oils exhibited antibacterial activity with varying magnitudes: nineteen showed activity against one or more bacteria. Cinnamon, lime, geranium, rosemary, orange, lemon and clove showed maximum activity against all the bacterial species tested, whereas aniseed, eucalyptus and camphor failed to inhibit any of the tested strains.

Both Gram-positive and Gram-negative bacteria were sensitive to the essential oils, with *Staph aureus* sensitive to fourteen oils. In general, cinnamon oil showed significant inhibitory effect against bacteria giving a zone of inhibition of 20.8 mm. Moderate effects were seen in lime, clove and lemon oils.

Based on the zone of inhibition screening, seven of the original twentyone essential oils: cinnamon, clove, geranium, lemon, lime, orange and rosemary, that had been identified as having antibacterial activity, then had their minimum inhibitory concentrations determined.

MICs for the seven oils revealed that cinnamon oil had the greatest antibacterial activity, with MIC values ranging from 0.8% to 3.2%, followed by clove oil with MIC values ranging from 1.6% to 6.4%. The other oils showed moderate MIC values. In this study cinnamon, clove, geranium, lemon, lime, orange and rosemary oils exhibited the strongest activity against selected bacterial strains.

It is interesting to note that lemon oil produced good results in this study, in marked contrast to results obtained by other researchers.

Bulgaria
Microorganisms of interest to the veterinary industry
In Bulgaria,[24] twelve essential oils were tested for their inhibitory activity against fourteen microorganisms of veterinary interest. The specified essential oils they tested were:

- common thyme (*Thymus vulgaris*)

- clove (*Syzygium aromaticum*)

- cinnamon (*Cinnamomum aromaticum*)

- marjoram (*Origanum marjorana*)

- tea tree (*Melaleuca alternifolia*)

- clary sage (*Salvia sclarea*)

- peppermint (*Mentha piperita*)

- lemon (*Citrus limonum*)

- lemongrass (*Cymbopogon citratus*)

- grapefruit (*Citrus paradisi*)

- oregano (*Origanum vulgare*)

- mandarin (*Citrus reticulata var. madurensis*)

The fourteen microorganisms used included *Staphylococcus aureus* ATCC 25923. The researchers noted interesting inhibitory effects against the bacterial and yeast isolates taken from animals. MICs varied from 0.8% to

2%. Zones of inhibition varied from 12 mm to more than 20 mm. Thyme, cinnamon, peppermint, lemongrass and oregano oils inhibited all organisms at 2.0%. Good antimicrobial activities were exhibited by lemongrass, clary sage and peppermint oils. Lemon, grapefruit and mandarin oils did not show antimicrobial activity against the microorganisms.

The researchers concluded: "In our study cinnamon, oregano, lemongrass and thyme exhibit the strongest activity against the selected strains with veterinary interest."

For further information
Hundreds of research papers have been published on the antimicrobial activity of essential oils and readers wishing to know more can do an internet search by going to Google Scholar and typing 'antimicrobial essential oils for MRSA' into the search bar. The abstracts are always free, occasionally the entire paper is also free, but usually the publisher makes a charge for the research article.

Chapter 10
Other Ways to Combat MRSA

Phage therapy

Phage therapy, pronouced either like sage or barge, is not a new system of killing bacteria, but one that has been in place since 1919. Although its origins were in Europe, by the 1930s, phages were being produced and marketed by a few large pharmaceutical companies in the USA. The popularity of phage therapy to cure bacterial diseases continued until antibiotics were introduced in the 1940s. Across Eastern Europe however, phage therapy continued to be used to great effect. It is still widely employed in Russia, Georgia and Poland, where extensive scientific research has been undertaken. Today, phage therapy is undergoing fresh research in several countries: the US, UK, India and other parts of Western Europe, where university microbiology departments are conducting *in vitro* trials with phages in the hope of finding an alternative to broad-spectrum antibiotics. One of the UK's leading researchers[1] into phage therapy says: "We have come a long way in our understanding of phage therapy since a damning report ... in 1934[2] effectively closed the door on bacteriophage therapy in the West. These viruses have been pivotal in the development of modern molecular biology and in addition, those countries that persevered with phage therapy have accumulated many decades of clinical experience. Utilising these two bodies of knowledge, it should be possible to revisit the concept of phage therapy in the West and to have a reasonable expectation of success, provided we have an appreciation of the limitations of phage use."

Bacteriophages (phages) are viruses that specifically target bacteria and cannot infect mammalian cells. Each phage is specific to a particular bacteria, so there will be a phage to kill *Staphylococcus aureus*, a phage to kill *Streptococcus*, a phage to kill *Salmonella*, a phage to kill *E. coli*, and so on. As each phage is specific to one particular bacterium, it means that the body's good bacteria, the intestinal flora, is not damaged. This is of great benefit to a sick person as the immune system remains intact. The unique quality of using phages over antibiotic therapy is that only the targeted bacterium is killed. There is no possibility of resistance being transferred to surviving bacteria, as happens when antibiotics are used, as there are no survivors. If we were to think of different bacteria as having a specific colour and that *E. coli* was, for example, the colour 'orange' then once the *E. coli* phage was adminstered it would seek out and destroy only the 'orange' bacteria, leaving all the other colours of bacteria intact. Phages multiply at the site of infection, which in the case of *E. coli* would be the intestinal tract. Once in place the phages multiply until all targeted bacteria have been killed. From a single bacterial cell, in excess of a hundred new phage virus particles may be liberated and each of these is able to go on to attack a new bacterial cell. These infection cycles have the potential to continue until all susceptible bacterial cells have been killed.

Phage therapy would seem to offer the prospect of a cure for bacterial infections that are currently outwitting antibiotic therapy, and without any of the side effects, such as diarrhoea, which often accompanies antibiotic treatment. However, the downside, according to Thomas Hausler, author of a book on phage therapy,[3] is that they are more difficult to administer than antibiotics as the physician needs special training in order to correctly prescribe and use phages. A precise diagnosis must be obtained in advance of prescribing phage therapy. A 'broad-spectrum' phage to completely replace broad spectrum antibiotics does not exist at present. However in Georgia, home of phage therapy, a cocktail of phages, known as a 'pyophage' is being used with success to treat a broad range of pathogens.[4] One of their most important phages is a highly virulent monoclonal staphylococcal bacteriophage active against 80% to 95% of *Staph aureus* strains, including MRSA. This phage mixture, which is effective against *staphylococci, streptococci, P. aeruginosa*, and *E. coli*, is used to treat burn wounds, osteomylitis, skin infections, eye and ear infections and infected wounds, including those containing multiple resistant *S. aureus*. Commercially, this phage composition is blended with the antibiotic ciprofloxacin, and used in a wound dressing product, called 'PhagoBioDerm'.[5]

Allicin: from garlic (*Allium Sativum*)

Everyone knows that garlic is 'good for you' and garlic cloves are eaten in various ways and quantities throughout most, though not all, of the world. Garlic cloves contain many beneficial compounds. Research[6] as far back as the 1940s, revealed that the major medicinal compound obtained from garlic is allicin, a powerful antibacterial. Allicin does not occur naturally in garlic. It is only present and active when fresh garlic is chopped, cut or crushed, allowing the sulphur compound alliin (pronounced alli-in), to mix with the enzyme allinase. These two compounds are stored in separate compartments within the garlic clove and only when the structure is ruptured do the two substances come into contact and form allicin. Fresh allicin is unstable and breaks down quickly when heated, completely losing its medicinal properties when cooked. Commercially available allicin (diallyl thiosulfinate) has now been stabilized by a patented process[7] and can be obtained by both consumers and medical practitioners.

As with many foods, there will be a few people with an intolerance, and garlic is no exception. Ironically, it is the allicin compound within garlic that can cause an allergic reaction, although this is relatively rare.

Microbiology research with allicin

In 2004, researchers[8] from two London microbiology departments conducted trials using a stable aqueous extract of allicin against thirty isolates of MRSA that had already shown a range of susceptibilities to mupirocin. Results showed that 82% of the strains had full or partial resistance to mupirocin but that all strains were sensitive to, that is to say inhibited by, the allicin preparation. When the allicin concentrations were increased, all MRSA isolates were killed. Other research conducted between 1999 and 2002, has looked at the mode of action[9] of allicin and how this contributes to its biological activity and the antibacterial activity[10] of garlic extracts against MRSA.

Silver

Crude silver was used to heal infections as far back as 69 BC, as even then it was known to control the spread of infection and to prevent meat from spoiling. Silver was used throughout the Greco-Roman Empire and Hippocrates, the father of medicine, taught his students that silver healed wounds and controlled disease. The healing properties of silver nitrate was described in the physicians' pharmacopoeia of the time.

Although a popular form of medicine, one side effect from the treatment can be discolouration of the skin, as the overuse of silver can cause a condition known as Agyria. The name is taken from the chemical symbol for silver, Ag. Once the skin turns a blue-grey colour, the process cannot be reversed.

In the late 1800s, a chemist[11] found that silver could be diffused through a liquid to make a solution. He coined the term 'colloidal' for it, from the Greek word '*kolla*' which means glue-like, although as it was not a true solution, it became known as a 'sol'. A few years later, a Swiss botanist[12] working with soft metals such as silver, found them to be antimicrobial when in the form of a hydrosol, and he coined the term oligodynamic. Several researchers during the first half of the twentieth century increased the understanding of silver's capability and created many medicinal silver-based products. Millions of people around the world, notably within the United States, were treated with silver ions. This trend continued until the widespread introduction of antibiotics in 1940.

Fresh research into the use of silver as a biocidal agent began in 1970, under the direction of NASA. University scientists[13] were able to achieve a significant biocidal effect, with kill rates within four hours, when working with silver ions. Now, in the twenty first century, silver is being re-evaluated as an antimicrobial in the light of increasing numbers of antibiotic resistant infections.

Silver can be chemically bonded to a doorknob, or painted surface etc., so that when bacteria are detected, the silver compound releases silver ions, killing all microbes that come into contact with it. Silver has been used in several innovative ways:

- as a paint additive providing a non-toxic, silver-based coating for hospital air ducts so that when bacteria are detected, the silver compound releases silver ions to the surface, killing microbes for the life of the product.
- in hand soap and washing powder.
- as a coating for washing machine drums.
- for wound dressings.

Silver research with MRSA

As silver is an inorganic material, it has withstood the bacterial resistance that has dogged antibiotics, and as silver is a natural material it does not cause problems in the environment when discharged from the body, unlike antibiotics and many other medications which are not environmentally compatible. One US research team[14] says: "Silver kills microbes by interacting with multiple binding sites that are unlike those used by organic antibiotics; the use of silver is therefore unlikely to promote antibiotic resistance." From the emerging realisation that antibiotics were unable to overcome the problem of bacterial resistance, and in particular MRSA, silver has regained some respect from the scientific and medical professions. By the end of the first decade of the twenty first century there were several pharmaceutical companies producing wound dressings that incorporated silver ions/nanoparticles.

In 2007, a team of researchers[15] conducted microbiology trials with several bacteria including *Staphylococcus aureas*, where zone of inhibition tests were carried out using a nanocrystalline silver and a commercially available silver dressing. The objective was to determine the antimicrobial activity of silver-containing dressings on wounds affected by biofilm. Results varied between dressings and microbes, with zone of inhibition for the *Staphylococcus aureas* being 2.6 mm to 6 mm.

Further research in 2007,[16] looked at whether there was any danger of silver, when utilised as a wound dressing, leading to bacterial resistance. The researcher evaluated other people's research procedures and measurements, and noted that different silver products released silver at different rates. He concluded: "the clinical incidence of silver resistance remains low, and emergence of resistance can be minimised if the level of silver ions released from products is high and the bacterial activity is high."

Recent research[17] with nanoparticles of silver looked at the potential for toxicity in the human body. Nanoparticles of silver work by releasing silver ions and by penetrating cells, which is exactly what an effective antimicrobial agent should do. The research team was able to demonstrate that nanoparticles of silver also penetrate mammalian cells. Inside the cell a process of oxidisation takes place whereby silver nanoparticles release silver ions, increasing toxicity. The silver nanoparticles are being incorporated into creams, deodorants and wound dressings, leading to concerns by some scientists that further research is needed before product safety can be established. Nanotechnology is a controversial subject, not only in medicine, but in many industries.

Big pharma

Several large pharmaceutical companies are looking for novel molecules to help mankind in its quest to combat infectious diseases. At the same time, some chemicals that were thought to be effective are now being re-evaluated in the light of fresh research. Triclosan was hailed as a cheap and effective antibacterial agent and although it can be effective in killing bacteria on surfaces like table tops, chopping boards and other surfaces (including the surface of the skin), some researchers have found that it leaves a residue. Some bacteria, including MRSA, survive in this residue and build a resistance. There is also an environmental concern as 60% of US rivers and streams contain triclosan in their sludge. The manufacturers[18] of triclosan are now investigating a selection of Australian essential oils as potential antimicrobials.

In summary

Essential oils were used to combat infectious diseases long before the introduction of antibiotics. Garlic, honey, silver and phage therapy were also employed to promote health and to combat infectious diseases. Throughout history anyone wounded in battle or through an accident, would be vulnerable to infection setting in. Although dangerous, having an infected wound was not necessarily a death sentence, nor should it be now. Back then many natural products were found to be effective. What differentiates the two eras is that we now have scientific evidence to prove why and how these products work against bacteria, whereas in the pre-antibiotic era there was scant scientific evidence. In general, antimicrobial products were used empirically, as knowledge of observable effects was passed down from generation to generation, or written up in herbals and medical compendiums. Then, as now, the key to a successful outcome was to treat early, not to wait for the bacterial growth to reach critical mass and invade the bloodstream. Once in the bloodstream MRSA is so much more difficult to treat, needing intravenous antibiotic treatment in order to save the life of the patient. Seventy years ago the old saying 'a stitch in time saves nine' would have been quoted. Today we would interpret this as 'prevention is better than cure'.

Part Three
APPENDICES

Nothing written about in Part Three is intended to take the
place of professional medical advice.

Appendix I
Facts & Figures

Microbes versus Humans

Number on Earth

Microbes:	50,000,000,000,000,000,000,000,000,000,000
Humans:	6,000,000,000

Mass in metric tons

Microbes:	50,000,000,000,000,000
Humans:	300,000,000

Generation time

Microbes:	30 minutes
Humans:	30 years

Time on Earth in years

Microbes:	3,500,000,000
Humans:	4,000,000

Source: Schaechter M. et al. Microbiology in the 21st Century. Where are we and where are we going? ASM, 2004. **www.asm.org**

Bacteria multiply by simple division, making a copy of their single chromosome and giving it to the new one. In laboratory conditions bacteria can double in number in twenty minutes, but take longer in and on human beings as bacteria have natural predators (intestinal bacteria for example), and only double once every twelve to twenty-four hours. They live in clusters, or families, and can do no harm as singletons. Millions are needed to produce enough toxins to cause disease. One hundred thousand billion (100,000,000,000,000) live on the skin and in the intestinal tract of a human being.

Antibiotic life lines

1929	Penicillin	discovered
1942	Penicillin	introduced
1947	Penicillin	resistance began
1947	Chlor-tetracycline	introduced
1960	Methicillin	introduced
1960s	Methicillin	resistance began, mid 1960s
1970s	Methicillin	widespread resistance by late 1970s
1964	Vancomycin	produced but not used owing to toxicity
1987	Ciprofloxacin	introduced
1990s	Vancomycin	brought into use in mid 1990s
1996	Vancomycin	first resistance noted
2000	Linezolid	introduced
2001	Linezolid	resistance noted in isolated cases

The time it took for MRSA to spread across Europe

1961	UK (MRSA first noted)
1965	France
1968	Denmark
1974	Ireland
1975	Switzerland
1978	Greece
1980	Belgium
1986	Netherlands

The Netherlands have the lowest incidence of MRSA in Europe. They had twenty-five years advance notice and were able to implement stringent proposals in hospitals. Every patient entering hospital is assumed to be an MRSA threat and placed in a specially built isolation ward. Only after swabs are negative is the patient admitted to the general hospital.

Europe-wide levels of MRSA resistance by end 2010

Malta	55%	UK	30%
Cyprus	55%	Other European countries	29% - 1%
Greece	40%	Norway	0% +
Ireland	33%	Holland	0% +

MRSA strains in the United States

Type Number:

USA 100	USA 200	USA 300	USA 400	USA 500
USA 600	USA 700	USA 800	USA 900	USA 1000
USA 1100	USA 1200	Brazilian*	Iberian*	

*these two clones are also responsible for 90% of MRSA outbreaks at the largest teaching hospital in Portugal.

Similarity of different MRSA strains in North America

USA 300 and USA 500 are similar

USA 400 and USA 700 are similar

USA 400 and USA 800 are similar

USA 1100 and USA 200 are similar

USA 100 is unique, lacking in similarity to any other strain

USA 600 is unique, lacking in similarity to any other strain

Work undertaken on strain typing shows close similarity of CA-MRSA in USA, Diversilab, Durham, North Carolina, USA.

Analysis of animal MRSA from dogs & cats in the UK

Epidemic strain EMRSA-15	95.4%
Epidemic strain EMRSA-16	1.6%
OTHER	3.0%

In addition:

- There are currently no vaccines available, although such products are reportedly in development stage.

- It can take around ten years and an average investment of one to two billion US dollars to bring a new antibiotic to the market.

- 235,000,000 doses of antibiotics are prescribed every year in the USA: 50% are not needed.

Reasons for Antibiotic Resistance

Some of the following are now considered history. Others are still very current.

No control over the sale of penicillin when first available

When penicillin was first manufactured in the USA in 1944, it was not a prescription drug, and continued to be available without a doctor's advice until the mid 1950s. It was marketed as a miracle cure and sold throughout the US in over the counter products such as creams, lotions and throat lozenges.

Misuse of antibiotics

- When antibiotics are prescribed unnecessarily: for viral conditions, for a minor ailment that would have 'run its course' but there is patient demand, by a doctor to hurry the patient out of the surgery.

- When antibiotic administration is delayed in critically ill patients.

- When broad spectrum antibiotics are used indiscriminately, or when narrow spectrum antibiotics are used incorrectly.

- When the dose of antibiotics is lower or higher than appropriate for the specific patient.

- When the duration of antibiotic treatment is too short or too long.

- When antibiotic treatment is not streamlined according to microbiological culture data results.

In surgery, when used as a prophylactic: "Many surgeons seek to compensate for poor hygiene conditions in their operating theatre or wards by employing routine prophylaxis use of antibiotics on uninfected patients 'just in case' ...

this results in excessive antibioic use and is certainly counter productive."
WHO report 1982.

When antibiotics are freely available
There is no control over purchase of antibiotics in many developing countries, where they can be bought as easily as sweets or cigarettes. Poorer citizens of the United States, unable to afford to visit a doctor, may opt to purchase the cheapest available antibiotic from an internet company when they, or a family member, are unwell.

Antibiotic use in agricultual animals
Antibiotics were routinely fed to cattle, pigs and other livestock in order to increase growth and prevent disease: disease often caused by unsanitary factory farming methods. Although many countries have banned the use of antibiotics to promote growth, and have created laws whereby only a veterinary surgeon can prescribe antibiotics for specific reasons, others continue to feed massive amounts of antibiotics to animals as a prophylactic. This allows them to legally add antibiotics to the animal feed. Animals have been given the very same antibiotics that are needed by humans to combat disease.

A serious consequence of the bad practice of feeding antibiotics to animals means that human consumers are eating meat containing traces of antibiotics. Whatever is consumed ends up in the waterways and is eventually piped into peoples homes. Almost all the water we drink, use for cooking, shower or bathe in, contains traces of antibiotics.

Evolutionary intelligence
Bacteria have evolved, and in doing so, developed not only clever defense mechanisms against being killed by antibiotics, but have also developed sophisticated means of attack, like the PVL strains of MRSA that attack and kill leukocytes, a vital part of the human immune system. Recent research with phenol soluble modulins (PSMs), is pointing to another evolutionary step: that CA-MRSA with PSMs can cause a cytokine storm.

Risk Factors

Risk factors are not universal and will vary from country to country. Risk factors also vary between healthcare-associated MRSA and community-associated MRSA. There are major differences between the strains of MRSA circulating in healthcare facilities and the strains found outside in the community. Generally, CA-MRSA responds to a wider range of antibiotics than does HA-MRSA, but can sometimes be very fast acting, causing fatalities in a matter of days.

Only a very few antibiotics are capable of killing MRSA once it has invaded the body and the patient has been diagnosed with bacteraemia. Preventing the progress of MRSA from colonisation to infection is the key to reducing morbidity and mortality caused by MRSA.

Risk factors for HA-MRSA

Being admitted to hospital

Whatever the age, the mere fact of entering hospital for an invasive procedure, whether hip replacement, plastic surgery or setting a broken bone, puts the patient at risk of contracting an MRSA infection. Being cut open, followed by the need for catheters and canulae, all create openings in the body, giving bacteria the potential to invade. Medical error has to be considered *Staphylococcus aureus* is a faculative aerobe (it can live without air) and when it gets into surgical wounds that are then closed, it can cause internal infections. Furthermore, any acute infectious disease such as influenza will lower the immune system, making the patient more vulnerable to opportunistic bacterial diseases.

It is estimated that in the UK, one in twenty people going into hospital will pick up an infection, MRSA being just one. Because these infections result in a longer hospital stay for the patient, the number of infected patients on any one day will be closer to one in ten.

Elderly and Frail

The elderly population of many developed countries are often required to move back and forth from their nursing home to a hospital. Nursing homes take care of the elderly with chronic health conditions, but when an acute problem presents, such as a fall or influenza, the elderly person will usually be admitted to hospital. For many elderly citizens these transfers happen on a regular basis. HA-MRSA moves effortlessly from hospital to nursing home and back again to hospital.

MRSA has been found in the oral cavity of several age groups, but most frequently in people of seventy years or older, with dentures also found to be colonised. A risk factor for oral carriage of MRSA among older people in long-term care is related to repeated antibiotic use and poor nutrition.

Babies and young children

When young children are hospitalised it is generally because of a serious health problem and/or a need for surgery. The immune system will be challenged by the illness itself, the surgery, the anaesthesia, and prescribed drugs; any one of these can weaken the immune system making the young patient more vulnerable to becoming infected with MRSA.

Broken Skin

Other risk factors include having a break in the skin where bacteria may enter, and this includes anyone suffering from eczema, as they could contract MRSA whilst visiting an elderly relative in a nursing home just as easily as when they are in hospital as an in-patient.

Community-associated MRSA

Outside of healthcare facilities, MRSA mainly manifests in the form of skin infections, causing swelling or growth, from a small pimple to a lump the size of a chicken's egg. Occasionally it causes a flesh eating disease in which tissue begins to die off, necessitating surgery to remove the decayed flesh. The amputation of an arm or leg may become necessary to prevent infection spreading to other parts of the body.

What to look for

A bump or infected area on the skin that may be:

- Red

- Warm to the touch

- Swollen

- Painfull

- Full of pus or other drainage

If you or someone in your family has these signs, especially with a fever, cover the area with a bandage and see your doctor.

Information from **www.cdc.gov**

A number of conditions and situations appear to increase the risk of contracting CA-MRSA infections and the following lists have been taken from advisory organisations. The USA currently experiences the highest number of CA-MRSA cases, and many of the following risk factors, at the moment, are specific to the US. CA-MRSA is on the increase in Europe.

Risk factors for CA-MRSA

In no particular order:

- Participation in contact sports. Most at risk are football players, wrestlers and basketball players, both professional and student.

- Sharing of towels or razors in sports facilities.

- Sharing of hot-tubs / jacuzzis.

- Busy gyms, particularly locker rooms, where there is a moist, sweaty atmosphere. Moist, warm areas are a perfect breeding ground for bacteria.

- Shared exercise equipment, unless wiped down between users.

- Living in overcrowded conditions such as prisons.

- Military bases: cramped living quarters.

- Day care centres for the elderly.

- Poverty: people forced to live in cramped conditions and suffer lack of hygiene.

- Day surgery: which could include circumcision or cosmetic surgery.

- Dentistry: tooth extraction.

- Tattoos.

- Childbirth, as bacteria could be on the hands of midwife/gynaecologist.

- Having a weakened immune system: e.g. a person living with HIV/AIDS, anyone receiving chemotherapy, transplant patients.

- Living with chronic ailments such as diabetes, severe asthma or eczema.

- Intravenous drug users.

- A severe attack of influenza can leave a person vulnerable to bacterial invasion. CA-MRSA pneumonia appears to occur most commonly following an influenza-like illness and may have special relevence given the emergence of swine flu (H1N1 influenza). Most worrying is that more children than adults are affected by flu-MRSA. Flu-MRSA cases are often fatal.

- Highest infection rate is in people of 65 yrs or more.

- African Americans are affected at twice the rate as other Americans.

- Native Americans and Pacific Island peoples show raised vulnerability.

- Although swimming in the ocean is not classified as a risk factor, a team of researchers in Florida have determined that bacteria can survive in the waters off Florida, as skin cells are shed whilst swimming, and that MRSA could potentially be picked up by bathers.

- Travelling on public transport comes with risks as MRSA bacteria can live on floors, door knobs, handles, seats and benches, it is easy for the superbug to spread.

Risk for our animals

Researchers in the UK have assessed risk factors for MRSA in dogs and cats as:

- contact with human carriers,

- surgical implants,

- admitted to veterinary clinic for 2 days or longer,

- having had at least 3 courses of antibiotics.

Appendix IV
Before Going into Hospital

We used to believe that if we had to go into hospital, we would be in safe hands, that a hospital was a safe environment in which to get well. We now know that is not the case. Hospitals are institutions that may be understaffed, underfunded, improperly cleaned. But above and beyond those factors, hospitals are full of sick people. The concentration of pathogenic microorganisms is far greater in a hospital than in any other institution. Disinfectants are no longer routinely being used in hospitals, with cleaning detergents taking their place. Detergents clean visible dirt but lack the ability to kill microorganisms. When going into hospital, do not assume anything. Do not assume a hospital is a clean and sterile place. Do not assume your requests will be implemented. Do not assume there will be sufficient staff on duty to adequately take care of every patient; although hospital staff will do their best, they are often overworked and struggle to give the required care to all of the patients. A former Chief Medical Officer[1] issued the following guidelines:

Advice for anyone going into hospital

- Patients on wards should insist doctors and nurses clean their hands thoroughly before examinations and procedures.

- Medical staff should also avoid their breath going onto a wound during a dressing change, and nor should you exhale directly over your own open wounds, uncovered cannula or catheters, as you or the clinician may be colonised in the nose or throat. Wearing a facemask is advisable.

- Insist that the patient's phone, table and locker are cleaned with antiseptic before use. Ensure that any bathrooms are clean before use.

- Do not allow your wounds or vulnerable sites to be attended to whilst cleaning is being done, nor within one hour of its completion. Dust carries germs and should be allowed to settle before your wounds are uncovered.

- Never allow your wounds to be left uncovered even for the briefest time. The longer they are exposed the greater the chance of infection getting in.

- The most vulnerable areas of skin prone to bed sores and consequent infection are the buttocks, elbows and heels. At the slightest hint of soreness insist on the area being sanitised and treated as a matter of urgency. Do not delay as this is a major entry point for infection.

- Never put bare feet on the ward floor.

- Do not allow visitors to sit on your bed.

- Paper may harbour infection. Politely decline another patient's offer of the use of their reading matter; avoid offence by explaining why.

- Ask your relatives to take laundry home in a secure plastic bag and wash separately in a hot wash above 65°C, or with a disinfectant. MRSA can live in fabric for approximately 60 days and withstand lower washing temperatures.

- It is recommended that you wash with antibacterial soap and shampoo for at least three days before admission, especially prior to surgery, as this may prevent you being a carrier and infecting yourself and others. Make sure that the groin area, between the toes and any other folds of skin are thoroughly cleansed and dried.

- Take a supply of antibacterial soaps and antiseptic wipes into hospital with you. Use these until you are discharged.

- There are many proprietary antibacterial preparations which may well add to your safety and may prevent the spread of infection. Be aware, however, that use of these preparations may offer a modicum of protection but will not prevent you from contracting a hospital infection, as in order for them to be totally effective it is necessary for everyone in the hospital to adhere to high hygiene standards.

How MRSA is spread in hospitals

Skin to skin contact remains the main mode of transmission for MRSA and many other infections, and all hospitals now implement a strict protocol whereby nurses and visitors are reminded to wash, or use an alcohol gel on their hands when arriving and when leaving a ward. Many nurses carry alcohol hand sanitisers on their belts, as they are required to wash their hands before and after attending to every patient. It has been demonstrated that nurses cleanse their hands more frequently than doctors or consultants, which is worrying, as it shows that strict hygiene standards are not yet being achieved.

MRSA can live on hard surfaces for several days and in fabrics for many weeks; it can also be passed from person to person via medical equipment and has been detected on stethoscopes, blood pressure cuffs, doctors' mobile phones, pagers and pens. The screens around a bed could harbour MRSA, as skin cells shed by previous or other patient(s) in the ward will have settled. MRSA can also live on floors, door knobs, taps, seating, tables and other furniture, including the patient's bedside locker.

MRSA is airborne. As skin cells are shed on a daily basis, so MRSA hitches a lift and is spread around hospital wards and corridors with the movement of patients, staff and visitors. Anyone, whether medical staff, auxiliary staff or visitors will be breathing in whatever is in the air, which means that anyone could be temporarily carrying MRSA. Masks are not routinely worn as health guidelines for mask wearing are not mandatory, and it is the decision of each hospital trust whether or not guidelines are implemented. As yet there is insufficient proof that MRSA is transmitted in the breath of a healthy person, and only when evidence is conclusive will the recommended guidelines become standard procedure in every hospital.

Once epidemic MRSA is established in a hospital it cannot be eradicated, only contained. This is why hospital admission is now classified as a risk factor in contracting an MRSA infection. For patients entering hospital, MRSA can become a bigger threat to their health than the diagnosed condition that necessitated admission to hospital in the first place.

Patients awaiting elective surgery are assessed to see if they are carriers of MRSA bacteria as decolonisation prior to hospital admission is a key point in minimising the incidence of MRSA infections in hospitals. Patients are being given mupirocin antibiotic cream to put up their nose and chlorhexidine or triclosan solutions for use in the bath or shower, in the weeks before admission for surgery.

Decolonising

To be assessed as colonised means that large numbers of bacteria are living on the body and inside the nose, and to decolonise is to reduce those numbers to a manageable level, though not necessarily to eliminate them completely. Researchers[2] have found a dramatic difference in the quantity of MRSA colonising the nose, and amongst people tested, some had as few as three colonies whilst others had 15 million colonies.

Mupirocin is most frequently given to colonised pre-surgical patients. It is effective at removing *S. aureus* from the nose over a few weeks of usage, but relapses are common within several months[3], and bacterial resistance to mupirocin is rising. Chlorhexidine is given to decolonise body sites and this remains effective. It is what surgeons have used for 'scrubbing up' prior to theatre surgery for many years.

Before going for a pre-surgical assessment I would recommend selftreatment with diluted essential oils in the assumption that if there was colonisation, then you have the potential to reduce the number of colonies, and if you were not colonised then it will not do any harm. Bearing in mind that bacterial resistance to mupirocin is rising, my feeling is that it is better to err on the side of caution, and self-treat prior to being swabbed at the pre-surgical assessment. If your swabs come back positive for MRSA you will be given mupirocin and a topical antimicrobial and told to go home and decolonise. By using essential oils it is possible you will have cleared yourself and if your swabs are negative you will be admitted for surgery without delay. If the majority of pre-surgical patients were able to decolonise themselves by using essential oil dilutions, then mupirocin could be used less often. This would be a good thing and may reduce the rise in bacterial resistance to it.

People wishing to prepare themselves for pre-surgery assessment by using dilute essential oils can find details of how to make simple products and which essential oils to use, in *Essential Oils* appendix. Let's not forget that soap and water is still a valid way of removing bacteria. We are constantly becoming contaminated when we touch items that are also touched by other people, for example elevator buttons, door handles, shopping trolly handles etc., but basic hand hygiene allows us to decontaminate. However, anyone with a heavy build up of bacteria, occurring most often at any one of the following sites, will be classified as being colonised.

Body areas where swabs will be taken to check MRSA status

Inside the nose	Use 1% dilution of essential oil in jojoba (a liquid wax) or a seed/nut oil twice a day. This is especially important before going to bed as bacteria and other microbes have a perfect opportunity to multiply whilst we are asleep.
Throat	Gargle with aromatic water. Spit out. Do not swallow.
Armpits	Wash with aromatic water. After drying the area with clean paper towels/tissues, use a 1% essential oil dilution to gently spread over the area. Leave on the skin for one hour before wiping off excess and putting on clothes. During that hour only wear a loose fitting bath-robe.
Groin	As for armpits.
Perineum	As for armpits.
Hair	Wash hair with a tea tree shampoo at least three days prior to admission. Alternatively make your own antimicrobial essential oil shampoo.

Taking a bath with one of the antibacterial essential oils will help to lessen bacteria on the skin, but the concentration of essential oil to a bath of water is not strong enough to kill MRSA. As bacteria are known to double in number every 24 hours, use diluted essential oils everyday on each of the specified body areas where swabs will be taken to ascertain MRSA status. Most of the university trials with MRSA bacteria used a 5% dilution of essential oil but as these were *in vitro* tests, and did not take into account the possibility of skin irritation, my recommendation is to use a 1% dilution.

All of the essential oils in the trials described in Part Two of this book inhibited the growth of bacteria, whilst a few showed a complete bacterial kill. As long as decolonising treatment is taking place on a regular basis, there is every possibility that bacteria will be prevented from multiplying and may be reducing. My advice is to use your best efforts to reduce bacteria but if you find you are sensitive to an essential oil then stop using it, just as you would stop using a deodorant or cologne if you experienced an adverse reaction.

Currently, when a pre-operative patient is given mupirocin and chlorhexidene and sent home to decolonise, they are not given any advice about the spouse/partner they share a bed with. Should they avoid intimacy? Should the partner be decolonised also? Could the partner be recolonising them? How frequently should nightclothes be washed? Information is minimal at the present time and patients are seeking advice from MRSA help groups. Presume your partner is in contact with the same levels of bacteria as you are and have them decolonise at the same time. Wash bedding and nightwear at the highest permissible temperatures and/or add antibacterial silver products to the wash.

Other recommendations

- Buy antiseptic hand wipes from a pharmacy or superstore and try them out at home, to make sure that you like the way they feel on your skin, and that the aroma is pleasant. There is a wide variety of products currently on the market and you may prefer one that is botanical, with an aloe vera base rather than an alcohol base. If you enjoy using the product, you are more likely to use it regularly whilst hospitalised.

- Surface wipes are cheaper than hand wipes and are ideal for wiping down hard surfaces around your hospital bed. Ward bathrooms are not always cleaned frequently enough and surface wipes are most useful here.

- You may wish to make up your own essential oil spritzer that can be sprayed around your bed, creating a pleasant aroma and giving you some peace of mind. Details of how to use antimicrobial oils can be found in *Essential Oils* appendix.

- Continue to keep the inside of your nose free of MRSA colonisation. Wards are generally kept warm and dry, and the inside of the nose is likely to be dry. Lining the inside of the nostrils with a little petroleum jelly or jojoba (a liquid wax) may discourage multiplication of bacteria. A small amount of either can be applied to the inside of the nostrils on a clean fingertip or cotton bud.

- Consider taking along your own pillow and change of pillowcase.

- Remember that you are your best defence against acquiring MRSA. Get a relative to speak on your behalf if you are too weak to do so yourself.

- Essential oils: take in your favourites to make your section of the ward more pleasant. Used with discretion, the natural aroma of essential oils are unlikely to upset anyone else on the ward.

- Treat any cuts and abrasions with an antiseptic and keep covered with a suitable dressing. Take a packet of plasters in with you so that you can decide when a change is due.

- Buy some inexpensive slippers that are easy to put on, and keep them in a shoe bag in your locker. Slip them on before you get off the bed, and when getting back into bed, only remove them when you are seated. Put them, soles together, into the shoe bag and stow in the locker. If you accidentally walk barefoot on the floor, sanitise the soles of your feet with an antiseptic wipe before getting back into bed. Consider disposing of the slippers instead of taking them home with you.

- Aim for the highest standards of environmental hygiene even if you have to implement them yourself. The area around a patient's bed needs to be kept clean: this includes the table, locker and floor, and is especially important when wards are crowded, with beds sited very close together.

- Once you are home and recovering it is still important to keep up a strict hygienic regime to protect your wound and your health.

Do not be afraid to ask
Do not be afraid to complain

- Do not be afraid to monitor what is happening to you and around you, and speak up if you are concerned that something is not right.

- Contaminated dressings and cotton swabs should be immediately bagged up and safely disposed of by clinical staff. You should avoid contact with such items.

- Before a doctor uses a stethoscope on your bare skin you can ask that it be wiped with an antiseptic. The same applies to blood pressure cuffs: if it is going onto your bare skin you have a right to request that it be sanitised. You might like to keep your own antiseptic wipes at hand to enable fast and efficient sanitising of these items.

- When a dressing is being changed and the clinician is not wearing a mask, it is prudent to request that they refrain from speaking whilst in close contact with your open wound.

- Drips (cannula) should not be left in place for more than three days. Each time the integrity of the skin is breached there is an opportunity for invasion by pathogenic organisms and intravenous cannulation is the most common invasive procedure amongst hospitalised patients. Guidelines[4] stating that cannulae be removed/re-sited every 72 hours are not mandatory. This means that individual hospital trusts can choose whether or not to implement the guidelines. Alert staff if you notice any redness or soreness at drip sites. Every hospital has an Infection Control Team: ask to speak to a team member if you have concerns. Their job is to minimize the risk of infection.

- Always remember that should you fall ill with an MRSA infection whilst in hospital or within days of returning home, you may not get any sympathy from hospital management. It is extremely difficult for an MRSA victim to bring a successful lawsuit against a hospital. Postoperative patients are now routinely sent home after a couple of days, which is in sharp contrast to procedures a generation ago when patients were kept in hospital for 7 – 10 days. A wound may not show signs of inflammation until four days after an operation, and this makes it easier for hospital management to claim that the surgical site became infected in the patient's home environment.

Long, long ago

Joseph Lister, known as the father of antiseptic surgery, insisted on the use of carbolic acid to clean hospitals as it was a powerful phenol that killed germs. He had noticed that people often survived the trauma of an operation but died of what was known as 'ward fever'. Lister had read about Louis Pasteur's work with microbes and believed it was these microbes carried in the air that caused diseases to be spread in wards. People who had been operated on were especially vulnerable as their bodies were weak, their skin had been cut open, and germs were able to get into the body with more ease. Lister then developed his idea further by devising a machine that pumped out a fine mist of carbolic acid into the air of the theatre during operations. Post-operative deaths due to sepsis fell from 50% to 15%. Lister's protocol has been replaced by aseptic techniques in operating rooms and the prophylactic use of antibiotics. Although surgery is now safer than in Lister's day, with regards to ward hygiene there is much scope for improvement.

Appendix V

Essential Oils

What is an essential oil?

An essential oil is the fragrant, volatile part of a plant which is removed by a process of distillation. This involves passing high-pressure steam through the plant material so that the aromatic liquid is separated from it. As the steam cools and turns to water the essential oil floats on top and is collected. Essential oils are volatile liquids and as such they work in several ways. They are also extremely complex, being composed of scores of chemical constituents, which in combination, give each essential oil its unique qualities. Every time a volatile oil dissipates into our immediate environment it is drawn into the body every time we take a breath. When inhaled, essential oil vapours enter the lungs where they combine with oxygen. As the oxygen enters the bloodstream so too do the aromatic vapours, eventually circulating throughout the body.

Diluting essential oils in jojoba or a fatty oil makes them instantly suitable for massage into the skin, applying to the inside of the nostrils or rubbing onto areas of the body where swabs are taken for MRSA analysis. Many books have been written on the subject of aromatherapy and there is no shortage of information on how essential oils work, their use throughout history, and how to blend essential oils to create pleasant and effective personal care items. This book has focused on research which demonstrates a proven role for essential oils as valuable antimicrobials.

How do essential oils kill bacteria?

Essential oils can easily mix with, and travel through, fats and oils, but do not mix with water and will always float on top. They are therefore known as lipophilic (oil loving) and hydrophobic (water hating). Although much research has been carried out into the antimicrobial action of essential oils, less research has been undertaken into how essential oils act against bacterial cells. While the precise mode of action is still being investigated, it has been suggested in one research paper[1] that it is the lipophilic properties of essential oils that interferes with, or partly solubilises, the cellular membranes of bacteria, disrupting normal activity. Another research paper[2] has found that the hydrophobic nature of essential oils, and their components, is an important characteristic, which enables them to partition the lipids of the bacterial cell membrane and mitochondria, disturbing the cell structures and rendering them permeable and prone to leakage and death. The essential oil "might cross the cell membranes, penetrating into the interior of the cell and interacting with intracellular sites; critical for antibacterial activity."

How to handle essential oils

Because essential oils are volatile substances they will evaporate when exposed to the air, and therefore they must be stored carefully. As a rule of thumb, replace the cap on the bottle immediately after use, keep out of sunlight, and store in a cool place. Room temperature is fine but keep oils away from radiators and fires. Always keep out of reach of children, as essential oils are concentrated plant essences that could harm a child if swallowed or rubbed into the skin and eyes.

As essential oils are concentrated they should always, with a few exceptions, be diluted before use. Unless you are familiar with essential oils, I recommend that you begin by using just one essential oil so that you can judge how it works: decide if you like the aroma and monitor any adverse reactions. Once you are comfortable with using the single essential oil you could move on to using another oil, and then with blending essential oils.

How to dilute essential oils

To make a massage oil: the simplest way to make a 1% dilution is to buy a 100 ml bottle of jojoba oil or a seed/nut oil and take out a small amount: no more than half a teaspoon. Then add twenty drops of essential oil to the bottle. Replace the cap and tilt the bottle until the contents are mixed. Most commercially available essential oils come in darkened glass bottles with an integral stopper, which makes it easy to count the number of drops.

To make an aromatic water: add a drop or two of essential oil to a clean, lidded jar, then add an inch or two of water. As essential oils will not dissolve in water you will need to replace cap and shake the jar thoroughly in order to disperse the oil throughout the water before each use. Alternatively, buy a 500ml bottle of water; remove a capful of water to make it easy to shake the water/essential oil sufficiently to disperse the essential oil throughout the water. Add drops of essential oil and shake well.

Useful conversions to determine the dilution of essential oil in 100ml bottle of liquid

20 drops	= 1 ml	= 1% dilution
40 drops	= 2 ml	= 2% dilution
1 teaspoon	= 5 ml	= 5% dilution

The main ways of using dilute essential oils

- **Application to the skin:** essential oils dissolve easily in fatty oils such as sweet almond, sunflower or olive. These are known as base oils. I prefer the liquid wax, jojoba, as it does not oxidize (go rancid) and can be kept for a long period of time, but when making an essential oil dilution for immediate use, this need not be a consideration. When essential oils are diluted in a base oil they have many uses: general body massage, application to the inside of the nostrils and as part of a care plan for the treatment of a chronic wound.

- **For antiseptic cleansing:** add a drop or two of essential oil to a clean, screw-top jar then add an inch or two of water, preferably pure bottled water. Essential oils will not dissolve in water so cap the jar and shake thoroughly to disperse the oil throughout the water before each use. Other uses for aromatic water include: throat gargle, mouthwash or to clean the inside of the nostrils.

- **Bathing:** for an adult with normal skin, use between 2 – 6 drops of essential oil to a full bath of water. Agitate the water to disperse the oil before getting in the bath. Use fewer drops for the elderly and infirm as their skin could be more sensitive. For children or animals, it is advisable to consult with an expert, or one of the many informative books on aromatherapy, before using essential oils.

- **Vaporise:** to scent the air in a room you will ideally use a source of heat in order to cause evaporation of the essential oil, although you can put a drop or two on the corner of a pillow that does not come into contact with the skin. Place a few drops of an oil, or oils, into a small dish of hot water. Or, put a drop or two of essential oil onto a tissue and place on top of a hot radiator. Alternatively, you may prefer to purchase an aroma stone, an electrically heated device onto which you drip essential oils. The best method is to find an electric diffuser/nebuliser that sends the essential oil into the room without heating it. There are diffusers that work with a current of air to break the essential oil into smaller particles which are then diffused into a room. You may want to bear in mind that hospitals do not permit the use of candles or electrically operated diffusers.

- **Spritzer:** very simple to make and easy to use. Add aromatic water to a spray bottle. Shake well before each use. Aromatic water is heavier than air and will drop down immediately, so remember that anything spritzed will be a little damp for a few minutes. Use on curtains, wipeable furniture and bedding.

- **Shampoo:** add up to a maximum of 20 drops of antimicrobial essential oil to 100 ml non-perfumed shampoo.

Specific uses of dilute essential oils for decolonising and maintaining good health as referred to in *Before Going into Hospital* appendix

- **Application to the inside of the nose:** to keep the nostrils free of bacterial build up, use a 1% dilution of essential oil in jojoba. Most of the essential oils mentioned in this book could be used for decolonising the nose, the exceptions being the spice oils cinnamon and clove, lemongrass, thyme linalool and the citrus oils, as each is a little too irritant for the delicate lining of the nose. Choose an essential oil you really like as the aroma will be very noticeable until it wears off.

- **Cleansing a small wound or scrape:** to cleanse a small wound simply place one drop of your chosen essential oil into a lidded jar with an inch or so of water and shake vigorously. Or use a small bottle of spa water. Dip a cotton pad or a clean cloth into the aromatic water to cleanse the area around the wound, before cleansing the wound itself. Do not introduce a soiled pad into the water. Use as many fresh pads as necessary to clean the wound. Put all used pads into a small plastic bag. Seal and place in bin/trash. Twice a day is ideal.

- **Treating a chronic wound:** see *Wound Care* appendix for hygienic care plan and practical advice.

Treating your pet with essential oils

Treating a pet other than your own is against the law. Treating your own pet with essential oils requires a considerable amount of knowledge and a pet owner should always consult with their veterinarian if concerned about a pet's health. If you are colonised with MRSA and are worried about your pet being colonised, you should talk to your vet about treatment options. Bear in mind that a vet can only advise the use of essential oils if they have received training. Alternatively you can perform an internet search for 'aromatherapy vets.'

Animals of different species can have different reactions to an essential oil. As an example, cats are unable to metabolise phenols and therefore thyme essential oils should not be used on cats, although there is no such problem with dogs. Pets living in the homes of aromatherapists will undoubtedly be in contact with the vapours of many essential oils, without any adverse effects, and I am of course erring on the side of caution in referring the reader to a veterinary professional.

See *Resources* for recommended reading material and training courses.

From the very wide range of essential oils available to the public, I have selected a few of those with antimicrobial activity referred to in Part Two. Whichever essential oil is chosen it needs to be correctly diluted.

Recommended antimicrobial essential oils for wound care

- tea tree
- thyme linalool
- manuka

Recommended essential oils for wound cleansing

- lavender
- clary sage
- manuka
- agonis fragrans
- geranium
- lelechwa
- tea tree
- thyme linalool

Recommended essential oils for washing colonised body areas: armpits, groin, perineum

- lavender
- manuka
- geranium
- tea tree
- clary sage
- agonis fragrans
- lelechwa
- thyme linalool

Essential oils for general bathing

- lavender
- bergamot
- geranium
- manuka
- clary sage
- agonis fragrans
- lelechwa
- thyme linalool

Essential oils for spritzing or vaporizing and that are not for use on the skin

- cinnamon
- orange
- lemongrass
- lemon
- grapefruit
- thyme linalool
- or use any of the oils recommended in above lists.

Essential oils for making an antimicrobial shampoo

- tea tree
- geranium
- thyme linalool
- manuka
- lavender
- or any of the citrus oils

Essential oils recommended for nose or throat

- manuka
- agonis fragrans
- tea tree
- clary sage

Jojoba oil, although more expensive than fatty oils such as sweet almond and sunflower, is my preferred choice for application of dilute essential oil to the inside of the nose, as it coats the surface, forming a barrier.

Wound Care

Colonisation vs infection

According to the website of the Health Protection Agency, the definition of **colonisation** is when MRSA is living in the nose or throat, or on the skin of the following areas: armpits, groin or perineum, and yet is not causing a problem to the individual.

When MRSA causes an active **infection**, the wound is red, hot, inflamed and there may be discharge and pain. If the inflamed area around the wound is severe it may be called cellulitis. When bacteria eventually infect the bloodstream the condition is known as bacteraemia. Then there is a huge grey area: what defines a wound that will not heal? If a wound is not healing because bacteria is multiplying and keeping the wound open, is it **colonised** or is it **infected**?

Infection Control personnel I have spoken with admit it can be confusing. Clearly any wound, whether from trauma or from surgery, if not adequately treated, can lead to blood stream infection. It is a numbers game. If bacteria, and in particular MRSA, are permitted to grow unchallenged, the bacteria will eventually win. From a fresh wound to a blood stream infection progress is in this order:

- Contamination
- Colonisation
- Critical colonisation
- Critical mass – when the bacterial load is so great that it goes into the body and causes bacteraemia.

Note: Wound care is vitally important in order to prevent potential bacteraemia.

If a wound is not healing then it is being kept open by something, as it is the body's natural urge to heal. That something could be a material item such as a surgical swab, but most commonly it will be a mixture of microorganisms, including MRSA. Anyone experiencing the inconvenience of a wound that will not close, and who has very recently been hospitalised, is quite likely to have an MRSA colonised wound. When bacteria in a wound are killed, the body will close the wound: this is the innate healing capacity of the human body. Antibiotics used to be able to facilitate this function, but increasingly, it is multi-drug resistant bacteria that hold the balance of power, with wounds remaining open.

A small amount of *Staph aureus* in an acute wound is a good thing, as it acts as a guard against more dangerous bacteria getting in and causing problems whilst the immune system is mobilising its defenses. As a rule the immune system will take care of the microorganisms as part of the healing process. Bacteria in a wound become a threat to health when the immune system is unable to control the growth and the bacteria multiply to a dangerous level.

My recommendation for anyone with a wound is to consult their doctor as soon as a problem is noticed, and not wait until the wound is causing pain, inflammation or malodour. This section of the book is for people who wish to tend to their own small wounds. Large wounds should always be dealt with by a medically trained person. When taking care of your own wound the main points to consider are:

- Hygiene
- Removal of debris
- Use of an effective antibacterial agent
- Dressing the wound

Items to have to hand
- Small plastic bags: sandwich bags are an ideal size.
- A packet of cotton pads, the kind used for removing makeup.
- Paper kitchen towels or paper napkins.
- Individually wrapped dressings, available from pharmacies.

- A small glass bowl, scissors and tweezers.

- Antimicrobial essential oil.

- Alcohol hand wipes.

- Aromatic water, see *Essential Oils* appendix.

- You may wish to purchase disposable plastic/latex gloves.

- A small plastic tray used solely for the purpose of wound care.

- Choose a room and time of day where you can quietly concentrate on what you are doing.

Cover the plastic tray with kitchen paper or napkins. Onto the covered tray place a small stack of cotton pads, the small glass bowl to which you will add the aromatic water, alcohol hand wipes or antimicrobial essential oil for sanitising the scissors and tweezers. The cutting away of dead skin and removal of slough is known as debridement, and in a hospital or a clinic would be carried out by nursing staff. I include the option here for those people who, because of geography, transportation or other reason, are unable to visit a medical facility or be visited by a district nurse, or when it is not possible to get a prompt appointment at a clinic.

Choice of antibacterial agent

- **Manuka honey medical dressing:** if your choice of dressing is manuka honey, you will still need to clean up the wound before applying the sterile manuka dressing, following manufacturers recommendations.

- **Essential Oils:** if your choice is to use essential oils, then make up preparations in accordance with directions in *Essential Oils* appendix. Anyone unsure of the reaction of an essential oil on their skin may wish to err on the side of caution and begin by applying a diluted essential oil to the soles of the feet. This area of the body has the thickest skin and if any itching or discomfort is noted then either try another essential oil in a day or two, or choose a different treatment method.

- **Silver dressings:** are prescription–only for wound care.

Hygienic care and disposal of contaminated items

A very important factor in the treatment of MRSA colonised wounds is the correct disposal of wound dressings and contaminated items. Washing of hands before and after treatment is important, even if disposable gloves are worn. Soiled material should be carefully disposed of by placing in a plastic bag, tying securely, and taking to the trash can. Spritzing an essential oil around the room will help to remove floating skin cells and airborne bacteria. Or vaporise essential oils into the room, see *Essential Oils* appendix.

- Firstly, open a sandwich bag and fold down the top so that you make a bowl shape. This is where all of the soiled items should be put.

- It is important to remove any debris from a wound as dead tissue can harbour bacteria. Yellow pus will provide nutrition for bacteria, so its removal will discourage rampant growth. When a wound is constantly covered with pus (slough), it prevents the formation of new skin cells and can give off an unpleasant smell. A wound, free of debris, has the optimum chance of healing. Debride means to cut away and remove debris from a wound.

- Disinfect the scissors and tweezers with an alcohol wipe before and after use, or alternatively wipe items with tissue impregnated with a drop or two of antimicrobial essential oil.

- Wipe/cleanse the wound with aromatic water and cotton pads. Only remove dead tissue. Cut it as though you were trimming your nails. Use tweezers to carefully remove debris along with the slough, but without causing yourself pain. Everything removed should be put directly into the opened plastic bag.

Use padded dressings which have a non-stick layer over the pad, which ensures that the pad does not stick to the wound. It is important that the dressing is larger than the wound so that the sticky part of the dressing only comes in contact with healthy skin, and not any part of the wound or surrounding area treated with oil. A dressing will not adhere to oily skin.

A suggested care plan using above information

Monitor your body's response and only continue with wound care if you feel comfortable. **Discontinue if you experience discomfort.**

Every day until healing takes place: cleanse the wound with disposable cotton pads soaked in aromatic water, see *Essential Oils* appendix. Cleansing with aromatic water will be sufficient for fresh wounds. Cover wound with suitable dressing immediately after cleansing and applying dilute essential oil.

- **Day 1:** rub a 1% essential oil dilution into the soles of both feet.

- **Day 2:** as Day 1.

- **Day 3:** cleanse wound with aromatic water, pat dry and apply diluted oil to the perimeter of the wound using a cotton pad.

- **Days 4 to 6:** as Day 3 plus gently spread the 1% essential oil dilution over wound.

- **Day 7:** cleanse the wound with aromatic water but switch to a 5% essential oil dilution to apply to the perimeter of the wound using a cotton pad. Debride the wound if necessary.

- **Day 8 to 10:** as day 7 apply 5% essential oil dilution to the wound if you can still see signs of infection such as white or yellow pus.

- **Day 11 and onwards:** Monitor the wound. If healing is taking place, only change and dress the wound every third day. You will know if your wound is healing as it will look and feel better, and there will be no bad smell. Continue to clean and dress your wound, but leave longer between treatments as healing progresses. Only debride when necessary.

- **This is very cautious approach.** If you are familiar with, and know you are tolerant of, your selected essential oil then proceed at your own pace to treat your wound.

- **Only debride** if you can see dead tissue and slough. Soaking the wound in or with aromatic water for 30 minutes or more prior to treatment will make debridement easier.

- **Caution when changing wound dressings:** if the dressing has stuck to the wound do not force it off. Soak the dressing with aromatic water. Tea tree or lavender is recommended.

If the wound is on foot/ankle or lower arm you could soak the extremity in a bucket containing aromatic water. Buy a plastic bucket specifically for wound care, and keep it sanitised.

If the wound is somewhere on the body where it cannot be soaked in a bucket of water, then soak a washcloth in aromatic water and apply over the old dressing. Leave in place for at least 30 minutes or until the old dressing can be easily removed.

Daily care:

- cleanse wound with aromatic water
- apply dilute essential oil
- dress wound

Weekly care:

- debride if necessary

It is quite likely that medical personnel will be dismissive of/frown upon a patient undertaking their own wound care. But I firmly believe that when it comes to the wellbeing of our own body(ies) we need to take more responsibility. There is a dearth of viable alternatives to topical antibiotics, and as a consequence many people are suffering the inconvenience and pain of living with a chronic wound caused by heavy MRSA colonisation.

Extra Reading

Superbug: nature's revenge

By GEOFFREY CANNON, Virgin Publishing Ltd., 1995.
Written in the early days of MRSA, this book has great insight and is full of information, both interesting and technical.

Plague Time: how stealth infections cause cancers, heart disease and other deadly ailments

By PAUL W. EWALD, The Free Press: division of Simon & Schuster, Inc., 2000.
An interesting book. The author likens the evolution of antibiotic resistance to Sisyphus of Greek mythology, who was condemned by Zeus to eternally push a rock uphill only to have it roll down again before reaching the hilltop. His thinking is that if we always had access to several new, narrow spectrum antibiotics we would constantly be challenging evolving bacteria, rather than being at its mercy.

Methicillin-resistant *Staphylococcus aureus*: A primer for dentists

Paper by R. MONINA KLEVENS et al., Journal of American Dental Association, 2008. A guide for dentists and/or people concerned with the possibility of picking up an infection during dental procedures.   **http://jada.ada.org**

Evaluating the Safety of Antimicrobial New Animal Drugs with Regard to their Microbiological Effects on Bacteria of Human Health Concern

FDA: The Food and Drug Adminstration, have a website with many interesting pages and downloadable PDFs, such as the above, that outlines a recommended approach for assessing the safety of new veterinarian antimicrobial drugs with regard to their microbiological effects on bacteria of human health concern.   **www.fda.gov/AnimalVeterinary**

IDSA: First Guidelines for Treatment of MRSA

MRSA has an enormous clinical and economic impact, and clinicians often struggle with the management of these infections. These guidelines provide a framework to help clinicians determine how best to evaluate and treat patients with both uncomplicated and invasive infections caused by MRSA. Many papers can be accessed at: **www.idsociety.org**

MRSA in hibernation

New strategies to apply antibiotics more effectively to hibernating bugs have been developed by researchers at the University of Hertfordshire. Details can be found at: **www.medicalnewstoday.com.** Type "MRSA in hibernation" into the search bar.

www.veterinarynursetrainingonline.org has links to dozens of articles of relevance to MRSA in animals.

Appendix VIII
Organisations

Around the world groups of people and individuals have set up organisations to address specific health concerns, each one hoping to make a difference by regulating or raising awareness in the efficient use of antibiotics, surveillance of antimicrobial resistance, better health care for minority groups and MRSA control. These organisations join the established agencies and colleges in providing relevant information.

EUROPE

RUMA

Responsible Use of Medicines in Agriculture Alliance is a unique initiative involving organisations representing every stage of the "farm to fork" process, RUMA aims to promote a co-ordinated and integrated approach to best practice in the use of medicines.   **www.ruma.org.uk**

RVC

Royal Veterinary College, London, works closely with the Bella Moss Foundation to increase awareness of MRSA and impart practical advice on the management of MRSA for all involved in veterinary medicine.   **www.thebellamossfoundation.com**

HPA

The Health Protection Agency is an independent UK organisation that was set up by the government in 2003, to protect the public from threats to their health from infectious diseases and environmental hazards. Across the UK, a representative sample of twenty-six hospitals keep a record of all *Staphylococcus aureus*/MRSA bacteraemias. Each hospital sends isolates from MRSA patients to ARMRL.   **www.hpa.org.uk**

ARMRL
Antibiotic Resistance Monitoring & Reference Laboratory is responsible for the detection and surveillance of antibiotic resistance, forwards data to EARSS. **www.hpa.org.uk**

EARSS
European Antimicrobial Resistance Surveillance System was established in 1998 to monitor the prevalence of antimicrobial resistance throughout Europe. The central database is in the Netherlands. **www.ecdc.europa.eu**

IPS
Infection Prevention Society exists to promote the advancement of education in infection prevention and control for the benefit of the community as a whole, in particular by the provision of training courses, accreditation schemes, educational materials, meetings and conferences. **www.ips.uk.net**

ReAct
Action on Antibiotic Resistance is a coalition that links a range of individuals, organisations and networks around the world taking concerted action to respond to antibiotic resistance. The organisation campaigns for the appropriate use of antibiotics, and for improved hygiene in hospitals to ensure better infection control. Based in Sweden. **www.reactgroup.org**

United States

IDSA
Infectious Diseases Society of America represents more than 8,600 infectious diseases physicians and scientists devoted to patient care, education, research, and public health. Their members care for patients with serious infections, including antimicrobial resistant bacterial infections, meningitis, pneumonia, surgical infections, HIV/AIDS, tuberculosis and influenza. **www.idsociety.org**

TFAH
Trust For America's Health is a non-profit, non-partisan organisation dedicated to saving lives by protecting the health of every community and working to make disease prevention a national priority. **http://healthyamericans.org**

SHEA

Society for Healthcare Epidemiology of America represents 1,500 physicians, infection control practitioners, and other healthcare professionals dedicated to maintaining the utmost quality of patient care and healthcare worker safety in all healthcare settings.　　　**www.shea-online.org**

STAAR

Strategies To Address Antimicrobial Resistance.

www.idsociety.org/staaract.htm

CSTE

Council of State and Territorial Epidemiologists is a professional association of over 1,500 members, representing the interests of public health epidemiologists for the 50 states, 6 territories, Puerto Rico and the Virgin Islands.　　　**www.cste.org**

NMQF

The National Minority Quality Forum is a non-profit health research and educational organisation dedicated to the elimination of health disparities. The Forum supports national and local efforts to eliminate the disproportionate burden of premature death and preventable illness in racial and ethnic minorities and other special populations.

www.nmqf.org

CDC

Centres for Disease Control, Atlanta, Georgia. The website gives general advice on MRSA and guidelines for both the public and healthcare professionals: "CDC is working with state and local public health authorities to monitor and investigate infections with MRSA, including pneumonias and other types of MRSA infections that occur in patients with influenza. CDC also acts as a technical advisor to state and local health departments and various professional organizations that are working to control MRSA."　　　**www.cdc.gov**

NARMS

National Antimicrobial Resistance Monitoring System is a national public health surveillance system that tracks antibiotic resistance in foodborne bacteria. The NARMS program was established in 1996, as a partnership between the US Food and Drug Administration (FDA), the Centers for Disease Control and Prevention (CDC), and the US Department of Agriculture (USDA).　　　**www.cdc.gov/narms**

APIC

Association for Professionals in Infection Control and Epidemiology is a body of professionals working to improve legislation, awareness and best practice in the control and treatment of infectious diseases **www.apic.org**

KAW

Keep Antibiotics Working. The Campaign to End Antibiotic Overuse includes concerned health, consumer, agricultural, environmental, humane and other advocacy groups with more than eleven million members, all working to reduce the growing public health threat of antibiotic resistance. **www.keepantibioticsworking.com**

UCS

Union of Concerned Scientists. This non-profit alliance of more than 200,000 citizens and scientists uses scientific evidence to lobby governments, corporations and consumers to act responsibly for the benefit of society. Their interest in antibiotic resistance focuses on reducing the use of antibiotics in food animals. The union encourages the public to get involved by writing to political representatives and signing petitions. **www.ucsusa.org**

US Government

50% of all antibiotics produced in the USA are for agricultural use. The US government is ushering in a bill to kerb antibiotic use in agriculture. For the latest developments go to **www.govtrack.us** and click on New Bills.

IDSA, TFAH, SHEA, CSTE, and APIC sent a joint letter to members of Congress, announcing their support for a new bill requiring national reporting of healthcare-associated infection rates to be contained within the healthcare reform.

International

APUA

Alliance for the Prudent Use of Antibiotics. Membership of this international group extends to more than a hundred countries. Through communication and education, the organisation seeks to promote improved use of antibiotics in order to prolong their long-term efficacy. **www.apua.org**

GAARD

The Global Advisory on Antibiotic Resistance Data is an initiative of the Alliance for the Prudent Use of Antibiotics (APUA), is the first project to assemble the data and findings from many of the world's largest antimicrobial surveillance systems into a comprehensive report on the state of antimicrobial susceptibility in the world today.   **www.apua.org**

Global Forum for Health Research is an independent, international organisation committed to demonstrating the essential role of research and innovation for health and health equity, benefiting poor and marginalized populations.   **www.globalforumhealth.org**

IFIC

International Federation of Inspection Control facilitates international networking in order to improve the prevention and control of healthcare associated infections worldwide.   **www.theific.org**

WHO

World Health Organisation publishes strategies for the containment of antimicrobial resistance. In the report 'WHO workshop on the containment of Antimicrobial Resistance in Europe', one section queried: "Perhaps MRSA should be a focus for concern over AMR and be considered an emerging infectious disease."   **www.who.int**

Products

Essential Oils

There are numerous websites supplying essential oils and many, though not all, carry a good quality range of essential oils for use by individuals and therapists. The following companies carry a high quality range of essential oils and have been chosen to distribute the newly available Benchmark thyme oil. For more information and direct links to distributors, visit the website. **www.benchmark-thyme.com**

UK

Aromantic Natural Skin Care
17 Tytler Street, Forres, Moray, IV36 1EL, Scotland.
Phone: + 44 (0)1309 696900 | Fax: + 44 (0)1309 696911
email: info@aromantic.co.uk **www.aromantic.co.uk**

Ireland

Atlantic Aromatics
9 Ardee Court, Bray, County Wicklow, Ireland
Phone: + 353 1 286 5399 | Fax: + 353 1 286 5414
email: david@atlanticaromatics.com **www.atlanticaromatics.com**

Canada

Green Valley Aromatherapy Ltd
4988 North Island Highway, Courtenay, BC V9N 9H9, Canada.
Phone: + 1 250 334-4836 | Toll Free: 1-877-572-7662 (Canada and US)
Fax: + 1 250 338-4835 | email: sales@57aromas.com
www.57aromas.com

USA

Ananda Apothecary
245 30th Street, Boulder, Colorado, 80305 USA | Phone: + 1 303 494 5561
email: information@anandaapothecary.com **www.anandaapothecary.com**

Aromatics International

9280 Mormon Creek Road, Lolo, MT 59847 USA
Phone: + 1 406 273 9833   **www.aromaticsinternational.com**

Earth Sweet Essential Oils

Crystal Baldwin, Golden, CO 80403 USA | Fax: + 1 303 642 3944
email: earthswt@aol.com   **www.earthsweetessentialoils.com**

Nature's Gift

316 Old Hickory Blvd., East Madison, TN 37115 USA
Phone: + 1 615 612 4270 (8:30 am - 4 pm Central Time Zone).
email: marge@naturesgift.com   **www.naturesgift.com**

Stillpoint Aromatics

415 Juniper Drive, Sedona, Arizona 86336 USA. Phone: +1 928-301-8699
email: info@stillpointaromatics.com   **www.stillpointaromatics.com**

Asia

Asia-Pacific Aromatherapy Ltd.

Room 1001, 10/F, Java Commercial Centre, 128 Java Road, North Point,
Hong Kong | Phone: + 852 2882 2444 | Fax : + 852 2882 5444
email: info@apagroup.com.hk   **www.aromatherapyapa.com**

New Zealand

Aromaflex

Trafalger St, Nelson, New Zealand | Phone + 64 3 545 6217
email: info@aromaflex.co.nz   **www.aromaflex.co.nz**

Making products with essential oils

Before attempting to make products containing essential oils you need
a good knowledge of essential oils and how to mix them with other
ingredients. I recommend two excellent books written by Kolbjorn
Borseth of Aromantic Skin Care Ltd: *Natural Spa Products – secrets of the
cosmetic industry revealed* and: *The Aromantic Guide to making your own natural
skin, hair and body care products.*   **www.aromantic.com**

Essential oil therapy for animals

Knowledge and experience of using essential oils is of paramount importance before treating an animal, and remember that it is against the law to treat an animal other than your own. To find a vet with a working knowledge of essential oils, an internet search will provide hundreds of sites from the input "aromatherapy vets". It is always advisable to speak with a veterinarian if your pet is unwell.

The Guild of Essential Oil Therapists for Animals (GEOTA) is the self-regulatory governing body in Essential Oil Therapy for Animals. GEOTA was set up to meet the overwhelming demand for people wanting to learn more about the use of essential oils with animals. GEOTA hold training programmes and their website has a list of therapists "qualified to educate pet owners in the safe use of essential oils on their own pets."

GEOTA

Horsehay Farm, Duns Tew Rd, Middle Barton, Oxon, OX7 7DQ, UK
Phone: + 44 (0)1869 349955 | Fax: + 44 (0)1869340969
email: geota@nhs4animals.com   **www.nhs4animals.com**

vetscpd@nhs4animals.com: email for information on training courses for veterinarians with an interest in using holistic medicine for animal health.   **www.nhs4animals.com/coursesforvets/index.htm**

An excellent book for pet owners on the safe use of essential oils is *Holistic Aromatherapy for Animals* by Kristen Bell, published by Findhorn-Forres, Scotland.

Other Products

Allicin

Allicin International Limited

Half House, Military Road, Rye, East Sussex, TN31 7NY UK
Phone: + 44 (0)1797 227959
email: norman@allicin.co.uk   **www.allicin.co.uk**

Silver Products

- **Silvatec hand soap,** incorporating silver ions, is available from several internet companies. The technical details can be found on-line. **www.giltech.biz/silvatec**

- **Silver impregnated plasters** are available from pharmacies, supermarkets and via the internet.

- **Silver wound care dressings** such as Acticoat by Smith & Nephew are only available on prescription via a healthcare provider.

- **Silverguard products** provide antimicrobial protection for textiles. A range of products for use in washing machines, or sprayed directly onto textiles, can be found at **www.silverguard.co.uk**

Manuka Honey

The internet has numerous sites selling manuka honey but for treating wounds it is advisable to purchase sterilised manuka wound dressings from a reliable company.

Comvita:

- **Medihoney:** medical grade manuka honey products including **Medihoney Apinate dressings** that are only available on-line.

- **Manuka honey:** in three strengths: UMF 10+, UMF 15+, UMF 20+.

- **Manukacare products,** containing manuka active 18+, are available in High Street stores across the UK.

Comvita UK Limited

Box 220, 5 High Street, Maidenhead, Berkshire SL6 1JN, UK
Phone: + 44 (0)1628 779 460 | email: info@comvita.co.uk
or info@comvita.com   **www.comvita.co.uk**
International: phone NZ: 0800 504 959 AUSTRALIA: 1800 466 392
                    www.comvita.co.nz | other countries www.comvita.com

Advancis:

- **Activon medical grade manuka honey:** a selection of manuka honey impregnated wound dressings are available online.

- **Actibalm:** applicator for treating lips, insect bites and scratches.

Advancis Medical Ltd

Lowmoor Business Park, Kirkby-in-Ashfield, Nottingham, NG17 7JZ

Phone: + 44 (0)1623 751500 | Fax: 0871 264 822

email: info@advancis.co.uk   **www.advancis.co.uk**

International: for distributors visit the contact section of the website.

Manuka Ratings

- When purchasing manuka honey, look for a reputable brand name.

- **The UMF trademark** is owned by the Active Manuka Honey Association (AMHA).

- **Active.** A grey area as some companies selling Active 10, Active 15 etc., do comply with standards similar to UMF but do not have a license from AMHA. Other companies using the word 'Active' may be selling honey of unreliable strength. Consumers should ensure that the activity of the honey they are purchasing is not solely peroxide activity.

- **MGO** is Methyl–glyoxal.

- **The Molan Gold Standard™** certification is available to honey manufacturers who meet the certification criteria set by Professor Peter Molan of the Honey Research Unit, Waikato University, New Zealand. This is a new rating.

Equivalent Ratings

- UMF 20 is twice as potent as UMF 10

- UMF 10 is equal to MGO 100

- UMF 20 is equal to MGO 400

- Active 10 is equal to UMF 10

Services

MRSA Support / Action Groups

www.mrsasupport.pwp.blueyonder.co.uk This site is a UK based forum for sufferers of MRSA or relatives of victims of MRSA. It facilitates communication with others in a similar predicament.

www.mrsaactionuk.net This website contains reliable information on the subject of MRSA. MRSA Action campaign for increased vigilance in the area of infection control, both inside and outside of hospitals, and regularly meet with government health bodies. Persons seeking advice prior to hospital admission can call the charity on + 44 (0)7762741114.

www.mrsaresources.com A US based web site set up and maintained for victims of MRSA infections focusing on education, awareness and support.

www.mrsanotes.com MRSA Notes is an offspring of MRSA Resources.

www.mrsa-forum.com is a US based support group forum where people can share their experiences of MRSA with other sufferers.

If you do not have computer access but would like to know what help is available on-line, your local public library will help you. Ask for the IT librarian. Often free lessons in using the internet are available, and there will be computer terminals you can use.

Microbiology tests to determine carrier status

Following discharge from hospital after an MRSA infection, you may be concerned about being an MRSA carrier, perhaps because you have elderly relatives or have young children or grandchildren. Or you may still feel

---

unwell, months after returning home, and suspect that you may not be free of MRSA. You may wish to have swabs taken and analysed so that you will know your status. If your GP dismisses your concerns, or says that the practice does not have the necessary funds to undertake such analysis, you can have swabs taken privately. The tests have to be carried out in a clinic, as swabs need to be correctly taken and sent for laboratory analysis. The London Clinic will take swabs from five body areas and give you a report. It is necessary to ring for an appointment and you would need a referral from your healthcare provider, should you wish to be seen by an expert. At the moment there are no clinics outside of London offering this service in the UK.

The London Clinic

20 Devonshire Place, London, W1G 9BW, UK
Phone : + 44 (0)20 7935 4444   **www.thelondonclinic.co.uk**

Wound healing

Chronic wounds that just won't heal are commonplace in people throughout the UK; MRSA is one of the many bacteria that can prevent a wound from healing. Sadly, there are no statistics being kept, which means that the numbers of sufferers are unknown. If MRSA is suspected, or if you have already been informed that your wound is colonised with MRSA bacteria and the prescribed treatment has not been effective, you can seek private assessment and treatment. People in the catchment area may be entitled to NHS funding. The clinic uses alternatives to antibiotics and has a high success rate, with wounds healing in approximately six weeks. They use a variety of effective, natural products.

The Wound Healing Centre

10 Gildredge Road, Eastbourne, BN21 4RL, UK
Phone: + 44 (0)1323 735588
Fax: + 44 (0)1323 737132   **www.woundhealingcentres.org**

Action Against Medical Accidents (AvMA)

AvMA personnel are available to give advice to anyone who has picked up Hospital Aquired MRSA. Initial advice is given on a telephone helpline, but more intensive/specialist support is available if required. It is not a walk-in service, so ring for an appointment. They also offer advice to people who have been bereaved by MRSA. Some of the services they offer are:

* Help with understanding medical terminology.

* An explanation of the processes available to persons seeking answers/ compensation after the death of a loved one. This allows the person to make an informed choice.

* Specialists can advise people whether or not they have a legal case. Legal cases are complex and expensive to instigate and pursue. Very few win their case, which can increase distress at a difficult time.

* A list of vetted, specialist solicitors.

Action Against Medical Accidents
44 High St, Croydon, Surrey, CR0 1YB, UK
Phone: 0845 123 2352 (10am – 5pm Mon - Fri)
Fax: + 44 (0)20 8667 9065   **www.avma.org.uk**

MRSA in animals

The Bella Moss Foundation (BMF)
Bella Moss was the first recorded case of death from MRSA in a dog in the UK. The foundation was set up by Jill Moss to raise awareness of MRSA in animals and to promote new research into MRSA and other serious infections in companion animals.

Their new **Animal MRSA Advice Service** will be an educational tool for lay people and veterinarians to learn more about resistant bacterial infections in animals.
email: info@thebellamossfoundation.com
www.thebellamossfoundation.com

www.veterinarynursetrainingonline.org A website set up for veterinary personnel as an offshoot of The Bella Moss Foundation.

www.pets-mrsa.com A forum, where questions and answers relating to MRSA in pets, can be found.

Glossary

Agar plate: a petri dish containing a growth medium (typically agar + nutrients) used to culture microorganisms.

Antagonist: something that reduces the activity of a substance.

Antibiotic classification: a **broad spectrum** antibiotic can be used against a variety of bacteria / fungi as opposed to a **narrow spectrum** antibiotic which is used to kill a specific microorganism.

Antimicrobial: a substance that kills or inhibits the growth of microorganisms such as bacteria, fungi, or protozoans.

Bacteraemia: the presence of bacteria in the bloodstream.

Bactericide / bactericidal: a substance with the power to kill bacteria.

Bacteriostatic: a substance that is powerful enough to prevent the growth of bacteria, although not powerful enough to kill off the bacteria.

Barrier nursing: also known as 'bedside isolation' when caring for a patient known or thought to be suffering from a contagious or infectious disease. The aim is to erect a barrier to the passage of pathogenic organisms between the patient and other patients or staff in the hospital.

Biofilm: a collection of bacteria or other microorganism in which they adhere to each other and/or a surface and then produce a slimy covering, effectively giving the bacteria a protective element against antimicrobials.

Broad spectrum: see antibiotic classification.

Camphoraceous: smelling of camphor.

Canula or cannula: a needle is inserted into a vein on the arm or back of hand, then pulled out leaving a flexible tube for the delivery of fluids.

Carrier / carriage: a person carrying MRSA is colonized without necessarily being affected by it.

Cellulitis: skin infection caused by bacteria, triggering severe inflammation of the connective tissue.

Chemotype: predominance of one chemical compound, either naturally occurring or created by hybridization.

Clone: a group of organisms, or cells, of the same genetic constitution as another, derived by asexual reproduction.

Chlorhexidine: a chemical antiseptic, both bactericidal and bacteriostatic, effective on Gram-positive and Gram-negative bacteria.

Clostridium botulinum: a bacterium that is sometimes found in honey.

Collodial solution: where particles are mixed in such a way that they remain evenly distributed in a liquid.

Colonised: to be carrying the MRSA bacteria. Common sites are: armpits, groin, perineum and inside the nostrils.

Commensal: common and benign bacteria living on and in humans. Cytokine storm: cytokines are components of the immune system and include interferons that trigger inflammation as a response to infections. Research is still being undertaken to accurately define a cytokine storm and it is thought that hormones are also involved. Under normal response mode, the immune system mounts a defence to fight off an invading pathogen e.g. influenza. A cytokine storm is an abnormally magnified/multiplied action of the immune response, which not only kills the pathogen but overwhelms the normal balance (homeostasis) of the body and kills the host.

Cytotoxic: quality of being toxic to cells. Can be either a product of the immune system or a chemical substance.

Endogenous: when a person with staphylococci spreads the bacteria from one part of their body to another part.

Endotoxin: poison produced by the death of bacteria, such as MRSA. In infected people, endotoxins cause fever and weaken capilliaries, causing fluid to leak into surrounding tissues which can cause a sudden drop in blood pressure, resulting in toxic shock.

Exogenous: when organisms are transferred from person to person by direct contact or via contaminated environment or equipment.

Exotoxin: poison released by bacteria that enters the bloodstream and causes serious problems throughout the body. Exotoxins are among the most poisonous substances known.

Faculative aerobe: an organism able to grow with or without the presence of oxygen.

Fusidic acid: an antibiotic that is used topically in creams and eye drops, but is only given internally in combination with other drugs.

Gram-negative / Gram-positive: In 1884, a Danish scientist called Gram experimented with bacteria, by adding a purple dye, leaving it overnight and then washing the bacteria with an inert liquid. The bacteria that stayed purple he called Gram-positive. The ones that washed out he called Gram- negative. All *Staphylococci* are Gram-positive, and *Streptococci* are all Gram- negative bacteria.

HAI & CAI: UK terminology, Hospital Acquired Infection & Community Acquired Infection.

HAI & CAI: US terminology, Hospital Associated Infection & Community Associated Infection. This terminology is now also being used in the UK.

H1N1: Hemagglutinin, Neuraminadase. Swine flu is H1N1.

Holistic: in alternative/complimentary medicine, refers to the treament of an individual by taking into account all aspects of their well-being, disease state, life sytle, diet, etc. and treating the person as a whole, rather than just treating the disease.

Holistic: in medical world, refers to treating a disease with multiple drugs and/or topical antimicrobials such as fusidic acid/chlorhexidene simultaneously in order to bombard the infection and save the life of the patient.

Hydrosol: a collodial solution.

ICU: Intensive Care Unit. The same term is used in both the US & UK.

INCI: International Nomenclature of Cosmetic Ingredients.

Inoculum / innoculum: the number of bacteria present on a petri dish at the beginning of a microbiology test, measured in logs.

Isolates: specific bacteria taken from patients' wounds, urine, etc. for use in microbiology tests.

Log: the short form of logarithm. Bacteria are grown on an agar plate (petri dish) until the bacteria have multiplied to a required amount. Log 3 would be a low inoculum of 1,000 bacteria per ml., Log 5 a medium inoculum of 100,000 bacteria per ml. Log 10 would be a very high inoculum of 10,000,000,000 per ml.

Loopful: a loop is a laboratory tool used to apply bacteria to an agar plate.

MBC: Minimum Bactericidal Concentration, smallest amount of substance needed to kill bacteria.

Malodour: a bad smell.

Mersa / Mursa: US terms for MRSA.

MIC: Minimum Inhibitory Concentration, smallest amount of substance needed to halt the growth of bacteria.

Microbes: bacteria (*Staphylococcus and Streptococcus*), viruses (influenza virus, chicken pox), fungi (*Candida albicans*). Sometimes newspaper articles refer to MRSA as a virus but this is incorrect.

Mupirocin: pseudomonic acid, a fermentation product produced by *Pseudomonas fluorescens* (NCIB 10586), a standard treatment for the carriage of MRSA.

Monoclonal: a group of cells produced from a single ancestral cell by repeated cellular replication.

NCTC: National Collection of Type Cultures, a library of micro-organisms.

Nanocrystalline: in a vacuum chamber, pure silver is bombarded with positive ions to liberate individual atoms. These silver atoms are then re-formed into new high-energy nanocrystalline structures.

Nanoparticles: are sized between one and one hundred nanometres. A nanometre is equal to one billionth of a metre.

Narrow spectrum: see antibiotic classification.

Necrosis: the death of tissue cells, which is now becoming more common in CA MRSA infections. The infection continues to spread through the body until all the infected tissue, or limb, is surgically removed. Streptococcal bacteria can also cause this type of damage.

Necrotizing fasciitis (NF): commonly known as' flesh-eating disease' is a rare infection of the deeper layers of skin and subcutaneous tissues. Historically, *Streptococcus* made up most cases but since 2001, it has been observed that *Staphylococcus aureus* was a major source of the disease. Without surgery and medical assistance, the infection rapidly progresses and eventually leads to death.

Nosocomial: healthcare-environment acquired condition.

Osmolarity/osmosis: ability of a substance, such as honey or salt, to draw water from an object.

Paradox: a statement that seems to be absurd or self-contradictory but may be true.

Pathogen / pathogenic: an infectious agent (or germ) such as a virus, bacteria, prion, or fungus that causes disease to its host.

Perineum: area between the anus and the genitals.

PICC line: Peripherally Inserted Central Catheters, used to deliver intravenous chemotherapy or antibiotics.

Prophylaxis: another word for preventative.

PSM: Phenol-Soluble Modulins, a family of protein toxins that are soluble in phenols and produced by CA-MRSA, and thought to be the cause of severe infections. Non-methicillin resistant bacteria are not found to produce PSMs. Although the toxins are produced in all MRSA strains, the more virulent CA-MRSA strains have a higher number of toxins.

PVL: Panton-Valentine Leukocidin toxin was originally discovered in 1894, but named in 1932 after the two scientists, Panton & Valentine who found the connection between it and soft tissue infections. The toxin kills leukocytes (white blood cells), an important part of our immune system. This particular toxin makes MRSA bacteria more deadly as it kills the leukocites which would normally defend the body against bacteria.

PVL MRSA: CA-MRSA with PVL toxins

Polymorphic: occurring in several or many forms or appearing in varying forms in different developmental stages.

Polymorphism: diversity occuring within biological populations, determined gentically or by environment.

Purulent: something that creates pus is called suppurative, pyogenic or purulent.

Quaternary ammonium: a powerful antimicrobial used in pre-operative disinfectants and soaps. Also commonly used in swimming pools to prevent a build up of algae over the winter months. Benzethonium chloride and benzalkonium fluoride are both quaternary ammoniums.

Sepsis: infection of a wound with bacteria resulting in localised pus. Blood poisoning.

Septicaemia: a life-threatening condition caused by a rapid build up of bacteria in the blood stream which overpowers the immune system.

Septic shock: a life threatenting condition when there is a dramatic drop in blood pressure as a result of septicaemia.

Sol: short form of hydrosol.

Solubilise: to make soluble, help to dissolve. An agent that increases the solubility of a substance.

Synergist: something that enhances the action of a substance, as when two or more essential oils produce a better result than any of the oils used singly.

Systemically: affecting the entire organism or bodily system.

TCP: brand name of a liquid used for disinfecting cuts and scrapes of the skin. Originally comprised of the chemical tri-chloro-phenylmethyliodosalicyl (hence its name) but reformulated in the 1950s to a mixture of phenol and halogenated phenols.

Topically/topical: medication applied to body surfaces such as the skin, eyes or mucous membranes.

Turbidity: when something is turbid it is muddy, thick, not clear.

Tween 20: a surfactant used in microbiology labs as either an emulsifier or as a washing agent.

Venturi effect: a combination of air pressure and velocity that creates lift off e.g. as when a plane takes off.

ZoI: Zone of Inhibition.

Zoonotic: a disease capable of jumping the species barrier. Technically, the transfer of disease from human to animal is anthroponosis, and animal to human is zoonosis. The terms zoonosis and zoonotic have beeen adopted for both modes of transmission.

References

Authors, institutions, papers, and publication are included. However, journal volume, pages and paragraph references have been omitted for brevity. Upon request the publisher will make all necessary corrections for the next imprint.

Part One – MRSA
Chapter 1   MRSA – World View

[1] Dr. Gro Harlem Brundtland, Director-General of WHO, July 1998-July 2003.

[2] New Scientist article originally published in the Lancet vol 365, 2005.

[3] Department of Microbiology and Infectious Diseases, Royal Perth Hospital, Australia. *Lecture given at the International Symposium on Staphylococcal Infections, Cairns Convention Centre, Cairns, Australia.* September, 2008.

[4] Smith J.M., Cook G.M., Department of Microbiology & Immunity, Otago School of Medical Sciences, University of Otago, N Z. *A decade of community MRSA in New Zealand.* Epidemiology and Infection, 2005.

[5] Professor Keiichi Hiramatsu. Juntendo University, Tokyo, Japan. 1997.

[6] Nanae A., Hori S., Department of Infection Control Science, Juntendo University, Japan. 2004.

[7] Kobayashi H., Japan. *National Hospital Infection Surveillance on MRSA.*

[8] Zhang R., Eggleston K., Rotimi V., Zeckhauser R.J. *Antibiotic resistance as a global threat: Evidence from China, Kuwait and the United States.* Laboratory research conducted at Faculty of Medicine, Kuwait University, Kuwait, 1999 – 2001.

[9] Park C. et al., Department of Internal Medicine, College of Medicine, the Catholic University of Korea, Seoul, Korea. *A survey of community-associated methicillin-resistant Staphylococcus aureus in Korea.* Journal of Antimicrobial Chemotherapy, 2008.

[10] Kim M.N. et al., Department of Clinical Pathology & Department of Internal Medicine (Infectious Diseases), University of Ulsan College of Medicine & Asian Medical Centre, Seoul, Korea and Department of Bacteriology, Juntendo Univesity, Tokyo. *Vancomycin-intermediate Staphylococcus aureus in Korea.* Journal of Clinical Microbiology, 2000.

[11] Seo Young Lee et al., Gachon Univesity Gil Hosptial, Incheon, Seoul, Korea. *A case of primary infective endocarditis caused by community-associated MRSA in a heathy individual and colonization in the family.* Yonsei Medical Journal, 2009.

[12] Udo E.E. et al., Department of Microbiology, Kuwait University, Molecular Genetics Research Unit, Curtin University of Technology, Perth, Australia. *Genetic*

Lineages of Community-Associated Methicillin Resistant Staphylococcus aureus in Kuwait Hospitals. Journal of Clinical Microbiology, 2008.

[13] Batkam N., Esener H. et al., Department of Infectious Diseases and Clinical Microbiology, Ankara Numune Education and Research Hospital, Ankara, Turkey. *American Journal of Infection Control,* 2008.

[14] Narezkina A., Edelstein I., Dekhnich A., Stratchounski L., Pimkin M., Palagin I., Institute of Antimicrobial Chemotherapy, Smolensk, Russia. *Prevalence of methicillinresistant Staphylococcus aureus in different regions of Russia: results of multicenter study.* Paper: 12th European Congress Clinical Microbiology and Infectious Diseases, Milan, 2002.

[15] Shittu A., Nubel U., Lin J., Gaogakwe S., Department of Microbiology, Obafemi University, Nigeria. *Characterisation of MRSA isolates from hospitals in KwaZulu- Natal province, Republic of South Africa.* Journal of Medical Microbiology, 2009.

[16] www.thestar.co.zo

[17] Dr Charles Lautenbach, an orthopaedic surgeon in South Africa, who has specialised in bone infections for over 30 years.

[18] Professor Guy Richards, Johannesburg Hospital.

[19] Mshana S.E. et al., Weill Bugando Medical College of Health Sciences, Mwanza, Tanzania. Tanzania Journal of Health Research, 2009.

[20] Mallick S.K., Basak S., Department of Microbiology, Jawaharlal Nehru Medical Centre, Wardha, India. *MRSA – too many hurdles to overcome: a study from Central India.* Tropical Doctor, The Royal Society of Medicine Press, 2010.

[21] Anbumani N. et al, Department of Microbiology, Sri Ramachandra Medical College & Research Institute (Deemed University), Chennai, South India. *Prevalence of MRSA in a tertiary referral hospital in Chennai, S.India.* Indian Journal for the Practising Doctor, 2006.

[22] Mohanty S., Kapil A., Dhawan B., Das B.K., Department of Microbiology, AIIMS, New Delhi, India. *Bacteriological and antimicrobial susceptibility profile of soft tissue infections from Northern India.* Indian Journal of Medical Science, 2004.

[23] Verma S. et al. *Growing problem of methicillin resistant staphylococci – Indian scenario.* India Journal of Medical Science, 2000.

[24] Nema S. et al., Choithram Hospital & Research Centre, Indore, India. *Emerging bacterial drug resistance in hospital practice.* Indian Journal of Medical Science, 1997.

[25] Deurenberg R.H., Vink et al. *The molecular evolution of methicillin-resistant Staphylococcus aureus.* Clinical Microbiology and Infection, 2007.

[26] Gertie van Knippenberg-Gordebeke.

[27] Stenham M. et al., Swedish Institute for Infectious Disease Control, Solna, Sweden. *Imported Methicillin-Resistant Staphyloccus aureus, Sweden.* Center for Disease Control Journal Emerging Infectious Diseases, 2010.

[28] Cercenado E. et al., Servico de Microbiologia, Hospital General Universitario Gregorio Maranon, Madrid. *CA-MRSA in Madrid, Spain: transcontinental importation and polyclonal emergence of PVL- positive isolates.* Diagnostic Microbiology & Infectious Disease, 2008.

[29] Holzknecht et al. *Changing Epidemiology of MRSA in Iceland from 2000 to 2008: a Challenge to current guidelines.* Journal of Clinical Microbiology, 2010.
[30] HPA – Local and Regional Services Management of PVL-*Staphylococcus aureus* Recomendations for Practice. www.hpa.org.uk
[31] Dr Angela Kearns, head of the Staphylococcal reference unit at the HPA, London, England.
[32] Professor Jeremy Hamilton-Miller.
[33] Survey headed by Dr Cooper of the National Institute of Health, 1977.
[34] Study headed by Professor Tomasz of the Rockefeller Institute in New York, 1994.
[35] GeneOhm, a company who have developed a diagnostic test that gives MRSA results in 2 hours. Quote from company spokesperson, 2007.

Additional information from:

- *The Antibiotic Paradox* by Stuart B Levy, MD. 2002
- *Superbug – Nature's Revenge* by Geoffrey Canon. 1995.
- Center for Disease Control (CDC), Atlanta, USA
- Johnson A.P. et al., Department of Healthcare-Associated Infection and Antimicrobial Resistance, Communicable Disease Surveillance Centre, HPA, Collindale, London, UK.

Chapter 3   MRSA in Animals

[1] Park, Yong Ho. Dept of Microbiology, College of Veterinary Medicine, Seoul University, Korea. *Epidemiology and origins of antimicrobial resistance in animals, 2007.*
[2] RUMA – Responsible Use of Medicines in Agriculture Alliance. Dr Tony Andrews is director and founder of the organisation, based in Hertfordshire, England.
[3] Dr David H Lloyd, Professor of Veterinary Dermatology, Royal Veterinary College (University of London) England. *Presentation at veterinarian seminar, UK, 2009.*
[4] IDEXX Laboratories, West Yorkshire, UK.
[5] The Bella Moss Foundation, www.thebellamossfoundation.com
[6] www.veterinarynursetrainingonline.org Set up to educate veterinary staff into the problems of MRSA and the best methods to counter the problem.
[7] The London Clinic.
[8] Rankin S. et al. *PVL toxin positive MRSA strains isolated from companion animals.* Veterinary Microbiology, 2005
[9] Dr Scott Weese, University of Guelph, Ontario, Canada. *The Second International Conference on MRSA in Animals.* London, England. Presentation, 2009.
[10] Shimizu A. et al. *Genetic analysis of equine MRSA.* Journal of Veterinary Medical Science, 1997.
[11] Christianson S. et al. *Comparative genomics of Canadian epidemic lineages of MRSA.* Journal of Clinical Microbiology, 2007.

[12] Weese J. et al. *Attempted eradication of MRSA colonisation in horses on two farms.* Equine Vet, 2005.

[13] Weese J. et al. *MRSA in horses at a veterinary teaching hospital: frequency, characterisation, and association with clinical disease.* Journal of Veterinary Internal Medicine, 2006.

[14] Dr Stuart Levy, Alliance for the Prudent Use of Antibiotics (APUA). Dr Levy is the author of *'The Antibioic Paradox'*.

[15] Devriese LA., Hommez J. *Epidemiology of MRSA in dairy herds.* Research in Veterinary Science, 1995.

[16] ST398

[17] The Ontario Veterinary College, Canada.

[18] Smith T.C. et al., Iowa University. *Isolation of MRSA from swine in the midwestern United States.* Journal of Infectious Dieases, 2006.

[19] Smith T.C. et al., Iowa University. *MRSA strain ST398 is present in midwestern US swine and swine workers.* PloS One, Public Library of Science, 2009.

[20] IDSA. www.idsociety.org

[21] Soil Association. *MRSA in farm animals & meat: a new threat to human health.* 2007.

[22] Bayer.

Additional information taken from:

- Rich, M. *Staphylococci in animals: prevalence, identification and antimicrobial susceptibility, with an emphasis on MRSA.* British Journal of Biomedical Science, 2005.

Chapter 4   The Evolution of MRSA

[1] Jevons P.M. *Celbenin - resistant Staphylococci.* British Medical Journal, 1961.

[2] Barrett F.F., McGehee R.F. Jr., Finland M. *Methicillin-resistant Staphylococcus aureus at Boston City Hospital: bacteriologic and epidemiologic observation.* New England Journal of Medicine, 1968.

[3] Schentag J.J., Hyatt J.M., Carr J.R., Paladino J.A., Birmingham M.C., Zimmer G.S., Cumbo T.J. *Genesis of methicillin-resistant Staphylococcus aureus (MRSA), how treatment of MRSA infections has selected for vancomycin-resistant Enterococcus faecium, and the importance of antibiotic management and infection control.* Clinical Infectious Diseases, 1998.

[4] Kluytmans J., van Belkum A., Verbrugh H. *Nasal carriage of Staphylococcus aureus: epidemiology, underlying mechanisms, and associated risks.* Clinical Microbiology Reviews, 1997.

[5] Daum R.S. *Clinical practice – Skin and soft-tissue infections caused by methicillinresistant Staphylococcus aureus.* New England Journal of Medicine, 2007.

[6] Herrmann D.J., Peppard W.J., Ledeboer N.A., Theesfeld M.L., Weigelt J.A., Buechel B.J. *Linezolid for the treatment of drug-resistant infections.* Expert Review of Anti-infective Therapy (Hospital Medicine Virtual Journal Club), 2008.

[7] Davis S.L., McKinnon P.S., Hall L.M. *Daptomycin versus vancomycin for complicated skin and skin structure infections: clinical and economic outcomes.* Pharmacotherapy, 2007.

[8] Hiramatsu K., Hanaki H., Ino T., Yabuta K., Oguri T., Tenover F.C. *Methicillinresistant Staphylococcus aureus clinical strain with reduced vancomycin susceptibility.* Journal of Antimicrobial Chemotherapy, 1997.

[9] Chang S., Sievert D.M., Hageman J.C., Boulton M.L., Tenover F.C., Downes F.P., Shah S., Rudrik J.T., Pupp G.R., Brown W.J., Cardo D., Fridkin S.K. *Infection with vancomycin-resistant Staphylococcus aureus containing the vanA resistance gene.* New England Journal of Medicine, 2003.

[10] Lina G., Piémont Y., Godail-Gamot F., Bes M., Peter M., Gauduchon V., Vandenesch F., Etienne J. *Involvement of Panton-Valentine leukocidin-producing Staphylococcus aureus in primary skin infections and pneumonia.* Clinical Infectious Diseases 1999.

[11] Boubaker K., Diebold P., Blanc D.S., Vandenesch F., Praz G., Dupuis G., Troillet N. *Panton-Valentine leukocidin and staphyloccoccal skin infections in schoolchildren.* Emerging Infectious Diseases Journal, 2004.

[12] Wang R., Braughton K.R., Kretschmer D., Bach T.H., Queck S.Y., Li M., Kennedy A.D., Dorward D.W., Klebanoff S.J., Peschel A., Deleo F.R., Otto M. *Identification of novel cytolytic peptides as key virulence determinants for community-associated MRSA.* Nature Medecine, 2007.

[13] Boyle-Vavra S., Daum R.S. *Community-acquired methicillin-resistant Staphylococcus aureus: the role of Panton-Valentine leukocidin.* Laboratory Investigation, 2007.

[14] Oliveira D.C., Tomasz A., De Lencastre H. *Secrets of success of a human pathogen: molecular evolution of pandemic clones of methicillin-resistant Staphylococcus aureus.* The Lancet Infectious Diseases, 2002.

[15] Schachter B. *Slimy business – the biotechnology of biofilms.* Nature Biotechnology, 2003.

[16] Beenken K.E., Dunman P.M., McAleese F., Macapagal D., Murphy E., Projan S.J., Blevins J.S., Smeltzer M.S. *Global gene expression in Staphylococcus aureus biofilms.* The Journal of Bacteriology, 2004.

[17] O'Neill E., Pozzi C., Houston P., Smyth D., Humphreys H., Robinson D.A., O'Gara J.P. *Association between Methicillin Susceptibility and Biofilm Regulation in Staphylococcus aureus Isolates from Device-Related Infections.* Journal of Clinical Microbiology, 2007.

[18] Mann N.H. *The potential of phages to prevent MRSA infections.* Research in Microbiology, 2008.

[19] Turos E., Shim J-Y., Wang Y., Greenhalgh K., Reddy G.S.K., Dickey S., Lim D.V. *Antibiotic-conjugated polyacrylate nanoparticles: New opportunities for development of anti-MRSA agents.* Bioorganic & Medicinal Chemistry Letters, 2007.

[20] Tacconelli E., De Angelis G., de Waure C., Cataldo M.A., La Torre G., Cauda R. *Rapid screening tests for meticillin-resistant Staphylococcus aureus at hospital admission: systematic review and meta-analysis.* The Lancet Infectious Diseases, 2009.

[21] Devriese L.A., Vandamme L.R., and Fameree L. *Methicillin (cloxacillin) resistant Staphylococcus aureus strains isolated from bovine mastitis cases.* Zbl Vet B (Zentralblatt Fur Veterinarmedizin Reihe B-Journal of Veterinary Medicine Series B-Infectious Diseases Immunology Food Hygiene Veterinary Public Health), 1972.

[22] Voss A., Loeffen F., Bakker J., Klaassen C., Wulf M. *Methicillin resistant Staphylococcus aureus in pig farming.* Emerging Infectious Diseases Journal, 2005.

[23] Rich M., Roberts L. *Methicillin-resistant Staphylococcus aureus isolates from companion animals.* Veterinary Record, 2004.

[24] Shopsin B., Kreisworth B.N. *Molecular Epidemiology of Methicillin-Resistant Staphylococcus aureus.* Emerging Infectious Diseases Journal, 2001.

Chapter 5   Microbiology Explained

[1] www.standardsuk.com for more information on British Standard testing methods; www.cen.eu for European Standard testing methods.

Bibliography:

• Carson C.F., Cookson B.D., Farrelly H.D., Riley T.V. *Susceptibility of methicillinresistant S.aureus to the essential oil of Melaleuca alternifolia.* Journal of Antimicrobial Chemotherapy, 1995.

• Carson C.F., Hammer K.A., Riley T.V. *Broth micro-dilution method for determining the susceptibility of E.coli and S.aureus to the essential oil of Melaleuca alternifolia (teatree oil).* Microbios, 1995.

• Cox S.D., Mann C.M., Markham J.L., Bell H.C., Gustafson J.E., Warmington J.R., Wyllie S.G. *The mode of antimicrobial action of the essential oil of Melaleuca alternifolia (tea tree oil).* Journal of Applied Microbiology, 2000.

• Doran A.L., Morden W.E., Dunn K., Edwards-Jones V. *Vapour–phase activities of essential oils against antibiotic sensitive and resistant bacteria including MRSA.* Letters, Applied Microbiology, 2009.

• Edwards-Jones V., Buck R., Shawcross S.G., Dawson M.M., Dunn K. *The effect of essential oils on methiciliin-resistant Staphylococcus aureus using a dressing model.* Burns, 2004.

• Hammer K.A., Carson C.F., Riley T.V. *In Vitro Activities of Ketoconazole, Econazole, Miconazole, and Melaleuca alternifolia (Tea Tree) Oil against Malassezia Species.* Antimicrobial Agents and Chemotherapy, 2000.

• Mann C.M., Markham J.L. *A new method for determining the minimum inhibitory concentration of essential oils.* Journal of Applied Microbiology, 1999.

• May J., Chan C.H., King A., Williams L., French G. L. *Time–kill studies of tea tree oils on clinical isolates.* Journal of Antimicrobial Chemotherapy, 2000.

• Pattnaik S., Subramanyam V.R., Kole C. *Antimicrobial and antifungal activity of ten essential oils in vitro.* Microbios, 1996.

Part Two – ANTIMICROBIAL ESSENTIAL OILS
Chapter 6   Tea Tree

[1] Penfold and Morrison. *Some notes on the essential oil of Melaleuca alternifolia.* Australian Journal of Pharmacy, 1930. Published in the British Medical Journal, 1937

[2] Southwell L.A., Hayes A.J., Markham J., Leach D.N., New South Wales Agriculture, Wollongbar Agricultural Institute, Centre for Biostructural & Biomolecular Research, University of Western Sydney, NSW, Australia. *The search for optimally bioactive Australian tea tree oil.* Acta Horticulture, 1993.

[3] Aspres N., Freeman S., Skin and Cancer Foundation Australia, Sydney. *Predictive testing of the irritancy and allergenicity of tea tree oil in normal human subjects.* Journal of Dermatology, 2003.

[4] Thursday Plantation. www.thursdayplantation.com

[5] Carson C.F., Riley T.V. *Safety, efficacy and provenance of tea tree (Melaleuca alternifolia) oil.* Contact Dermatitis, 2001.

[6] Penfold A.R. *The germicidal value of some Australian essential oils and their pure constituents.* Journal & Proceedings, The Royal Society of New South Wales, 1925.

[7] Williams et al. *A study of antimicrobial activity of oil of Melaleuca (tea tree oil): its potential use in cosmetics and toiletries.* Cosmetics, Aerosols and Toiletries, 1990.

[8] Williams L.R., Stockley J.K, Yan W., Home V.N. *Essential oils with high antimicrobial activity for therapeutic use. Combinations of tea tree and Manuka are being investigated for therapeutic use against MRSA.* International Journal of Aromatherapy, 1998.

[9] Carson C.F., Riley T.V. *Antimicrobial activity of the major components of the essential oil of Melaleuca alternifolia.* Journal of Applied Microbiology, 1995.

[10] Southwell I.A. *Tea tree constituents.* Hardwood Academic Publishers, 1999.

[11] Professor Gary French, et al., St. Thomas's Hospital, London, England. *Time/kill studies of tea tree oils on clinical isolates.* Journal of Applied Chemotherapy, 2000.

[12] The Australian Society for Microbiology, Perth, Australia. *Tea tree oil: the science behind the antimicrobial hype.* A Microbial Odyssey hosted Oct 1-5, 2001. The Lancet, 2001.

[13] Carson C, University of Western Australia, Perth. Paper presented at A Microbial Odyssey, 2001.

[14] Aspres N., Freeman S., Skin and Cancer Foundation Australia, Sydney. *Predictive testing of the irritancy and allergenicity of tea tree oil in normal human subjects.* Journal of Dermatology, 2003.

[15] Caelli M., Porteous J., Carson C.F., Heller R., Riley T.V., Department of Microbiology, Queen Elizabeth II Medical Centre, W Australia. *Tea Tree Oil as an Alternative Topical Decolonisation Agent for MRSA.* Journal of Hospital Infection, 2000. Reprinted in International Journal of Aromatherapy, 2003.

[16] Dryden M.S., Dailly S., Crouch M., Department of Microbiology and Communicable Disease, Royal Hampshire County Hospital, Winchester. *A*

randomized controlled trial of tea tree topical preparations, versus a standard topical regimen for the clearance of MRSA colonisation. Journal of Hospital Infection, 2004.

[17] Messenger S., Hammer K.A., Carson C.F., Riley T.V., School of Biomedical and Chemical Sciences, The University of Western Australia. *Assessment of the antibacterial activity of tea tree oil using the European EN 1276 & EN 12054 Standard Suspension tests.* Journal of Hospital Infection, 2005.

[18] Blackwood and colleagues. *Doctors test tea tree oil body wash for MRSA.* British Medical Journal: Infectious Diseases, 2008.

Additional facts taken from:

- Carson C.F., Cookson B.D., Farrelly H.D., Riley T.V. *Susceptibility of methicillin resistant staph aureus to the essential oil of Melaleuca alternifolia.* Journal of Antimicrobial Chemotherapy, 1995.

Chapter 7 Manuka

[1] Cooke A., Cooke M.D. *An investigation into the antimicrobial propeties of manuka & kanuka oils.* Cawthron Report 2, 1994.

[2] Williams L.R., Stockley J.K., Yan W., Home V.N. *Essential oils with high antimicrobial activity for therapeutic use.* International Journal of Aromatherapy, 1998.

[3] Karkenthal M., Reichling J., Geiss H.K., Saller R. *Comparative study on the in vitro actibacterial activity of Australian tea tree oil, cajeput oil, niaouli oil, manuka oil, kanuka oil & eucalyptus oil.* Pharmazie, 1999.

[4] Christolph F., Kaulfers P.M., Stahl-Biskup E. *A comparative study of the in vitro antimicrobial activity of tea tree oils with special reference to the activity of b-triketones.* Planta Medica, 2000.

[5] Christolph F., Stahl-Biskup E. *Death kinetics of staph aureus exposed to commercial tea tree oils.* Journal of Essential Oil Research, 2001.

[6] Christoph F., Kaulfers P.M., Stahl-Biskup E. *In vitro evaluation of the antibactericidal activity of b-triketones admixed to melaleuca oils.* Planta Medica, 2001.

[7] Courtney W.J. *Antimicrobial composition containing manuka oil and Australian tea tree oil.* Formed part of a patent application for a blend of the two oils against a range of bacteria, 2001.

[8] Sackett W.G. *Honey as a carrier of intestinal diseases.* Bulletin of the Colorado State University Agricultural Experimental Station, 1919.

[9] Dold H. et al. Zeitschrift fur Hygiene und Infektionskrankheiten, 1937.

[10] White J.W. et al. Biochimica et Biophysica Acta, 1963.

[11] Professor Peter Molan's chapter: *'Honey: antimicrobial actions and role in disease management'* from the book *'New Strategies combating bacterial infections.'* Edited by Iqbal Ahman and Farrukh Aqil, Wiley-VCH Verlag GmbH, 2009.

[12] Russell K.M. (M.Sc.) *The antibacterial properties of honey.* Thesis, 1983.

[13] Allen K.L., Molan P.C., Reid G.M., Waikato University. *Non-peroxide antibacterial activity in some New Zealand honeys.* Journal of Apicultural Research, 1988.

[14] Mavric E., Henle T., et al. University of Dresden, Germany. *Identification and quantification of methylglyoxal as the dominant antibacterial constituent of manuka honeys from NZ.* Molecular Nutrition Food Research, 2008.

[15] Adams C.J., Manley-Harris M., Molan P.C., University of Waikato, New Zealand. *The origin of methyloglyoxal in New Zealand honey.* Carbohydrate Research, 2009.

[16] Adams C.J. et al., University of Waikato, New Zealand. *Isolation by HPLC and characterisation of the bioactive fraction of NZ manuka honey.* Carbohydrate Research, 2007.

[17] Stephens J., Molan P.C. *The explanation of why the level of UMF varies in manuka honey.* The New Zealand BeeKeeper, 2008.

[18] Professor Peter Molan, Waikato University, New Zealand. *A survey of the antibacterial activity of some New Zealand honeys.* Journal of Pharmacy and Pharmacology, 1991.

[19] Bardy J., Slevin N.J., Mais K.L., Malassiotis A. *A systematic review of honey uses and its potential value with oncology care.* Journal of Clinical Nursing, 2008.

[20] Jenkins R.E., Burton N.F., Cooper R.A., Cardiff School of Health Sciences, University of Wales, Cardiff, 2009.

Additional information taken from:

- New Zealand Institute for Crop & Food Research Ltd.
- Malcolm H., Douglas, et al. Department of Chemistry, Plant Extracts Research Unit, New Zealand Institute for Crop & Food Research Ltd, University of Otago, PO Box 56, Dunedin, N.Z.
- Perry et al. *Essential Oils from NZ Manuka and Kanuka: Chemotaxonomy of Leptospermum.* Phytochemistry, 1997.
- www.mgomanuka.com
- Professor P Molan, Honey Research Unit, University of Waikato. *Finding how MGO gets to be in manuka honey.* New Zealand BeeKeeper, 2009.

Chapter 8   Thyme

[1] Thyme: The genus *Thymus.* Edited by Elisabeth Stahl-Biskup and Francisco Saez: "The first piece of evidence for adaptive variation concerns the geographical and localized distribution of chemotypes in *T. vulgaris* in southern France. Based on bulk samples of plants, it is clear that phenolic chemotypes dominate thyme populations in hot dry sites close to the Mediterranean sea, whereas non-phenolic chemotypes dominate sites further inland, particularly above 400m elevation." A study comparing 12 sites at low altitude with sites above 400m, found that above 400m there were no phenolic plants.

[2] In 1887, Chamberlain was the first researcher to attribute antibacterial properties to thyme in his research with typhus bacterium.

[3] Marsh, P.D. *Microbiological aspects of the chemical control of plaque and gingivitis.* Journal of Dental Research, 1992.

[4] Piccaglia Roberta, Marotti M., Giovanelli E., Deans S.G., Eaglesham E., University of Bologna. *Antibacterial antioxidant properties of Mediterranean aromatic plants.* Industrial Crops and Products, 1993.

[5] Patent application 'Natural Broad-spectrum antibiotic', 1998, WO9856395. Withdrawn in 2000.

[6] Cosentino S. et al. *In vitro antimicrobial activity and chemical composition of Sardinian Thymus essential oils.* Letters: Applied Microbiology, 1999.

[7] Rota M.C. et al., University of Zaragoza, Spain, Murcian Institute of Investigation and Agricultural Development, Murcia, Spain. *Antimicrobial activity and chemical composition of Thymus vulgaris, Thymus zygis and Thymus hyemalis essential oils.* Food Control, Elsevier Journal, 2007.

[8] Oussalah M., Caillet S., Saucier L., Lacroix M., scientists from three Canadian research centres. *Inhibitory effects of selected plant essential oils on the growth of four pathogenic bacteria.* Food Control, 2006.

[9] Nelson R., Department of Clinical Microbiology, Western Infirmary, Dumbarton Rd, Glasgow, UK. *In-vitro activities of five plant essential oils against MRSA and VRE.* Journal of Antimicrobial Chemotherapy, 1997.

[10] Oregon State University. *Best treatment identified to reduce deadly staph infections.* Presentation: American Society of Health System Pharmacists, 2007.

[11] Caplin J.L., Allan I., Hanlon G.W., School of Pharmacy and Biomolecular Sciences, University of Brighton, Brighton, BN2 4GJ, UK. *In vitro anti staphylococcal activity of a blend of essential oils from different chemotypes of thyme (Thymus species) compared to that of the essential oil of tea tree (Melaleuca alternifolia).* Unpublished.

[12] Caplin J.L., Allan I., Hanlon G.W., School of Pharmacy and Biomolecular Sciences, University of Brighton, Brighton, BN2 4GJ, UK. *Enhancing the in vitro activity of Thymus essential oils against Staphylococcus aureus by blending oils from specific cultivars.* International Journal of Essential Oil Therapeutics, 2009. www.ijeot.com

Chapter 9   Further Research with Essential Oils

[1] International Conference on Antimicrobial Research, ICAR2010 Valladolid, Spain. 3-5 November, 2010.

Lelechwa

[2] Kuki Gallmann: Gallmann Memorial Foundation, P.O. Box 63704, Nairobi 00100, Kenya. www.gallmannkenya.org

[3] Africa Botanica. www.africabotanica

[4] Munden D. and the Department of Industrial Chemistry, University of Surrey, UK, 1989.

AROMATHERAPY VS MRSA

[5] David Munden. *Patent of Invention WO2006087569: Antimicrobial Composition.*

[6] Matasyoh J.C., Kiplimo J.J., Kiplimo J.J., Karubiu N.M., Hailstorks T.P., Department of Chemistry and Department of Animal Health, Egerton University, Kenya, Department of Chemistry, Hampton University, USA. *Chemical composition and antimicrobial activity of essential oil of Tarchonanthus camphorates.* Food Chemistry, 2006.

Agonis

[7] Wheeler J.R., Marchant N.G. *Agonis fragrans (Myrtaceae), a new species from Western Australia.* Nuytsia, Western Australian Herbarium, 2001.

[8] Fragonia TM, The Paperbark Company, Harvery, W.Australia.

[9] Hammer K.A., Carson C.F., Dunstan J.A., Hale J., Lehmann H., Robinson C.J., Prescott S.L., Riley T.V. *Antimicrobial and anti-inflammatory activity of five Taxandria fragrans oils in vitro.* Journal of Microbiology and Immunology, 2008.

[10] Wollongbar Agricultural Institute, Wollongbar, NSW, Australia.

[11] Division of Microbiology and Infectious Diseases at Path West Laboratory Medicine, Nedlands WA, and the Microbiology and Immunology Discipline of the University of Western Australia, Crawley, Western Australia.

Essential oils and blends vs MRSA for the treatment of burns

[12] Professor V. Edwards-Jones, Buck R., Shawcross S.G., Dawson M.M., Department of Biological Sciences, the Manchester Metropolitan University, Manchester, UK. Dunn K., Burns Centre, Wythenshawe Hospital, Manchester, UK.

[13] Citricidal: a natural anti-viral, anti-bacterial, anti-parasitic and anti-fungal derived from grapefruit seeds.

[14] Flamezine™ prevented inhibition; impregnated Jelonet™ was less effective than impregnated Telfaclear™.

[15] Venturi: when a plane powers down a runway, it is the pressure of air under and over the wings in combination with speed that produces 'lift off '. This process is known as 'the Venturi effect'.

[16] Scent Technologies, Wigan, Lancashire UK. 01942 248383. The machine is for commercial use, treating an area the size of a tennis court in a few minutes.

[17] V. Edwards-Jones et al. *The effect of essential oils on methicillin-resistant Staphylococcus aureus using a dressing model.* Burns, 2004.

More research with antimicrobial essential oils

[18] Chao, Oberg et al., Department of Microbiology, Weber State University, Utah, USA. *Inhibition of MRSA by essential oils.* Flavour and Fragrance Journal, 2008.

[19] American Type Culture Collection (ATCC).

[20] Dorman H.J.D., Deans S.G. Aromatic and Medicinal Plant Group, Scottish Agricultural College, South Ayrshire, UK. *Antimicrobial agents from plants: antibacterial activity of plant volatile oils.* Journal of Applied Microbiology, 2000.

156

[21] Pattnaik S. et al. Regional Medical Research Centre, Indian Council of Medical Research, Bhubaneswar, India. *Antibacterial and antifungal activity of ten essential oils in vitro.* Microbios, 1996.

[22] Prabuseenivasan S. et al. Entomology Research Institute, Loyola College, Chennai, India. *In vitro antibacterial activity of some plant essential oils.* BMC Complementary and Alternative Medicine, 2006.

[23] Department of Microbiology, Christian Medical College, Vellore, India and Institute of Basic Medical Sciences (IBMS), Chennai, India.

[24] Department of Veterinary Microbiology, Infectious and Parasitic Diseases, Section of Microbiology, Trakia University, Stara Zagora, Bulgaria.

Chapter 10   Other Ways to Combat MRSA

Phage therapy

[1] Professor Geoff Hanlon, School of Pharmacy and Biomolecular Medicine, University of Brighton, East Sussex, England. *Bacteriophages: an appraisal of their role in the treatment of bacterial infections.* International Journal of Antimicrobial Agents, 2007.

[2] Eaton M., Bryce Jones S. *Bacteriophage therapy: review of the principles and results of the use of bacteriophage in the treatment of infections.* The Journal of the American Medical Association (JAMA), 1934.

[3] Thomas Hausler. *Viruses vs Superbugs (a solution to the antibiotic crisis).* Published by Macmillan, 2006.

[4] Eliava Institute, Tbilisi, Republic of Georgia.

[5] Markoishvili K. et al. Georgian Technical University, Tbilisi, Georgia. *PhagoBioDerm Research.* International Journal of Dermatology, 2002.

Allicin

[6] Cavallito C., Bailey J.H. *Allicin, the antimicrobial principal of allium sativum. Isolation, physical properties and antibacterial action.* Journal of American Chemical Society, 1944.

[7] Bennett N.J., Josling P.D., Cutler Dr R., Infectious Diseases and Pathology, School of Health and Bioscience, Department of Biosciences, University of East London. *Stabilised allicin – a unique natural antimicrobial agent.* European Journal for Nutraceutical Research, 2008.

[8] Cutler R.R., Wilson P. *Antibacterial activity of a new, stable, aqueous extract of allicin against methicillin-resistant Staphylococcus aureus.* British Journal of Biomedical Science, 2004.

[9] Miron T., Rabinkov A., Mirelman D., Wilchek M., Weiner L. *The mode of action of allicin: its ready permeability through phospholipid membranes may contribute to its biological activity.* Biochimica et Biophysica Acta, 2000.

[10] Cutler R.R., Townsend T., Sweeney D., Mukimbi E. Antibacterial activity of garlic extracts against MRSA and Gram Negative Rods. British Journal of Biomedical Science, 1999.

Silver

[11] Thomas Graham.

[12] Karl Wilhelm von Nageli.

[13] University of Wisconsin.

[14] AgION Technologies, Boston, USA.

[15] Percival S.L., Bowler P.G., Dolman J. *Antimicrobial activity of silver-containing dressings on wound microorganisms using an in vitro biofilm model.* International Wound Journal, 2007.

[16] Chopra I., Antimicrobial Research Centre and Institute for Molecular and Cellular Biology, University of Leeds, UK. *The increasing use of silver-based products as antimicrobial agents: a useful development or a cause for concern.* Oxford University Press on behalf of the British Society for Antimicrobial Chemotherapy, 2007.

[17] Chemists at the University of Helsinki. *Toxicity of antimicrobial silver in products can be reduced.* Colloid and Polymer Science, 2010.

Big pharma

[18] Ciba Speciality Chemicals Inc., Consumer Care Divison, Ciba, Switzerland.

Part Three – APPENDICES

Appendix IV Before Going into Hospital

[1] Sir Liam Donaldson. *10 Point Checklist: How to reduce your risk of catching MRSA and other Hospital Acquired Infections.*

[2] Mermel et al. *Who is at risk of MRSA? New study identifies, qualifies & characterizes its prevalence.* Journal Infection Control & Hospial Epidemiology, 2010.

[3] Coates T. et al. *Nasal decolonisation of S.aureus with mupirocin: strengths, weaknesses*

[4] www.clean-safe-care.nhs.uk. Type 'cannula' into the search bar.

Appendix V Essential Oils

[1] Soderberg T. et al., University of Umea, Sweden. *Toxic effects of some conifer resin acids and tea tree oil on human epithelial and fibroblast cells.* Toxicology, 1996.

[2] Trombetta D. et al. *Mechanism of Antibacterial Action of Three Monoterpenes.* Antimicrobial Agents and Chemotherapy, 2005.

About the Author

Maggie first became interested in alternative medicine back in the early 1970s when it was called 'fringe medicine'. Her involvement with essential oils began shortly afterwards and became the mainstay of her medicine chest during pregnancy, childbirth and the rearing of three children with all the usual childhood diseases.

She was one of the first UK published writers on the subject of aromatherapy. Her first book, *Aromatherapy for Women*, published in 1985, went on to become an international bestseller, selling in excess of 700,000 copies worldwide. Four other books followed, commissioned by mainstream publishing houses.

With the publication of *Aromatherapy for Women* in Japan, her partners there successfully introduced aromatherapy to the Japanese market. In 1989, Maggie was the first to speak on the subject, returning many times to lecture in Kyoto, Osaka and Tokyo. Her essential oil and herbal essence products created and led the market in Japan for more than 10 years. She was also instrumental in setting up the company which sells Tisserand oils but has not been involved since the late 80s.

Maggie has travelled extensively in pursuit of the best quality essential oils: working with growers on three continents. Based on practical experience of using essential oils to overcome serious chest infections picked up in India, Maggie began investigating the possibility that a combination of essential oils might be effective in combating multi-drug resistant infections.

This led to working with the MRSA Support group and successful trials with volunteers. Maggie was inspired to continue the research and worked with the University of Brighton to investigate the antimicrobial effects of essential oils against MRSA. Maggie established Benchmark Oils Ltd to raise investment for the long-term research and to help bring important laboratory discoveries into the public realm.

Maggie was born in 1950. A single mother since 1984, she has managed to juggle work commitments, book writing and motherhood. She lives in Sussex, South East England, has three children and three grandchildren.

www.benchmark-thyme.com